ON MY WAY

TO

THE CANCER MONUMENT

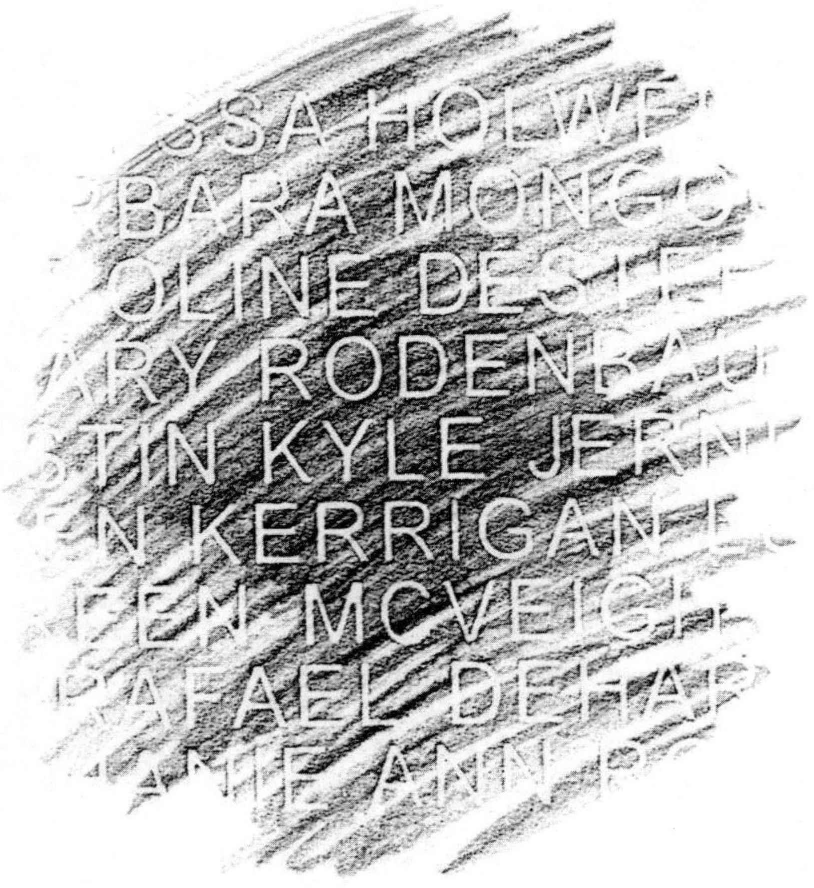

Graphic Composition by Annie Gough

"Every area of trouble gives out a ray of hope; and the one unchangeable certainty is that nothing is certain or unchangeable."

—John Fitzgerald Kennedy

ON MY WAY TO THE CANCER MONUMENT

A Monumental Cancer Battle Revealed

By Michelle Miller

Cancer Survivor, Monument Creator & Founder of

The Cancer Monument, Incorporated

With Sabra King

Foreword by Anna deHaro

On My Way to The Cancer Monument

Any opinions expressed herein, even those attributed to medical professionals, are not to be construed as medical advice. Consult your own physician for the appropriate diagnosis and treatment of cancer or any other disease or condition.

The Cancer Monument, it's architectural design, and logo are created by Michelle Miller and is a trademark of The Cancer Monument Incorporated. Any descriptive, media, or architectural likenesses, whether structural, temporary, artistic, or depictive of any sort are made with permission, guidance, and the written approval of Michelle Miller. Anyone claiming artistic design, or intellectual property ownership rights of The Cancer Monument, its methods, trade secrets, knowledge, or educational products whether published or unpublished is in violation of the law.

This book is part of the P.A.R.Q. Cancer Education Series. P.A.R.Q. Cancer Education Series is a 2004 copyrighted creation of Michelle Miller. The series is made exclusively and is licensed freely to The Cancer Monument Incorporated for the charitable purposes of achieving its mission statement through innovative educational media, products, and presentation services. Persons using P.A.R.Q. Cancer Education Series materials in a method not conducive to the author's intent are in violation of intellectual property laws. Materials shall not be stored, archived, edited, reproduced, distributed, or changed without the written authority the author. Fair Use and United States Copyright Act laws are permissable.

Printed in the United States of America
ISBN: 1-58752-254-3

10 9 8 7 6 5 4 3 2 1

Comments From Readers

"Michelle puts her heart and soul into everything she does and in so doing strengthens those around her in ways they may not even fully comprehend." *Laura Brougher, RN, BSN, OCN, Blood and Marrow Transplantation Services, Baylor University Medical Center, Dallas and Co-Founder of Cancer Together*

"Michelle writes with clarity and offers a resource filled with coping experiences and cancer related issues. I will give this book to patients, survivors, and their families who are going through the journey." *Audrey Thompson, R.N. OCN, Medical Center of Plano (Texas)*

"I had difficulty putting this book down. It should be a movie! This book is about a wonderful warrior, but it is so personal and displays so much that the public doesn't understand about how a person faces the diagnosis of cancer. The Cancer Monument is a wonderful way to honor those who have fought this dreaded disease." *Ginny Robinson, R.N., OCN, Medical Center of Plano*

"I love this story. Michelle's dream has to be shared with thousands." *Kathleen Bloom, Cancer Survivor, California*

"When I became a cancer warrior societal pressures on female beauty didn't really matter anymore. Growing up in Poland there was tremendous pressure to look like a runway model, or else be a failure. Michelle's cancer journey highlights the universal epidemic that links beauty with worth, and how having cancer can exacerbate the issue. Surviving cancer has made me realize that I'm okay no matter what." *Monika Mraovic, Melanoma survivor, Texas*

"Michelle's story appropriately motivates the patient to take charge of their health and healing. Her personal journey educates like a scholarly textbook but reads like a novel." *Maureen Kerrigan LupPlace RN, BS, OCN & Hodgkins' Lymphoma Survivor*

"Michelle's word imagery is fantastic. The need for The Cancer Monument became clear to me when she writes in Chapter 1: 'Wars are never won with just a single weapon. The same is true for the War on Cancer. Like artillery, The Cancer Monument is part of the solution.' " *Dena Plumer*

Acknowledgements

This book represents my 5-year journey to battle cancer, return to health, and life. In this brief time span there have been many challenges, unexpected losses, and unanticipated gains for me, and my family. However, in spite of this, there is much to celebrate. I am reminded that in all things teamwork is required. I also know that I never could have endured the battle without the love and support of many people. Whether in word or deed, each has reminded me of the existence of faith, love and the need for continuous hope. As a person, this has restored me. As a writer, I've been inspired. As a cancer monument visionary, I'm sustained by the truth of my mission and am grateful to the many talented people who have carried the torch of light and given their knowledge to the onward march of building a legacy - The Cancer Monument. There are not pages enough to express my thanks to:

My husband, Joey who is my reason for living
Rebecca & Paul Hartsfield, Shawn & Curtis Osmond, Stacey & Danny Vess
The Cancer Monument Board of Directors, Advisory Board and Volunteers
City of Allen government and Parks & Recreation Department: Mayor Steve Terrell, Peter Vargas & Allen City Council members, Tony Hill, Tim Dentler, Sue Witkowski
Dr. Edward Agura, M.D., Cancer Together, Laura Brougher, Baylor Hospital, Blood & Marrow Clinic
The National Marrow Donor Program
Dr. Denise Bannister, M.D.
Dr. Wendy Harpham, M.D.
Dr. Edward Gilbert, M.D.
Dr. Smith, M.D.
Dr. Dennis Birenbaum, M.D., Patients Comprehensive Cancer Center
Audrey Thompson; Allen & Plano Dialogue Support Group; Ginny Robinson, Oncology Nursing Society, Medical Center of Plano, Maureen LupPlace
Dr. Amanullah Khan; Cancer Center Associates; Trudy Benedict

Dr. Susan Williams McElroy, Associate Professor Economics & Education Policy, State University of Texas at Dallas, Douglas Kiel,

Ph.D., Professor of Public Administration and Political Economy, State University of Texas at Dallas,

KHYI 95.3 and KXEZ 92.1 Radio: Greg Patterson, Holly, Lou, and Hal, Timberwolf Press: Bill, Kurt, Jim, Rebecca, Tracy, & Carol; Sharon Mayer, Allen Chamber of Commerce

Mike Hathaway, Angie Alexander, Tempest Productions, The Valcik and Loney families, Our many others supporters: corporations, non-profit organizations, & Honoree families across the U.S.A, The Rodenbaugh Family, Danny McLarty, Kyle Feruguson, Ron Miller & Associates, Davis Munck, Chuck Bloom, Dena Plumer

Mike, Gloria, Ben, Shaun and LeSaan, Denise, Art Jennifer & Al, Carla Marion & KRLD 1080 AM, Jeff Elliot, Anna DeHaro, Clear Channel Radio Mix 102.9, KTVT CBS Channel 11-Dallas, Texas; Eileen Gonzales & KXII CBS Channel 12- Sherman, Texas; Ellen Sawko, Debbie Thomas, Allen American Newspaper, WFAA Channel 8; Dallas Morning News

Carrie Jackson, Cindy Patti, Karen Pierce, Connie Chaney, Linda Price & Laura Freer, Buddy, Aggie, Rowdy, Frank, and Mocha, Labrador Retriever Rescue of North Texas, Allen Animal Shelter, Dallas Chapter American Cancer Society, Dallas Junior Chamber of Commerce and to all who've consented to allowing their stories to be told in this book, I am grateful.

Photo of Michelle Miller by Joey Miller. Hair Design by Billy Humphreys.

Cancer Monument graphics by Image Technologies

Granite inscriptions by Reed Memorial / Granite Guys

Special Thanks

It's impossible to enumerate in a short space my gratitude to Sabra King. As professional writers know, there are many seen and unseen components that make a book. Many people are involved and not all are given credit. Multifaceted is the best way to describe a collaborator's unglamorous role, aside from the obvious technical requirements of writing, research, interviews, editing, endless re-writing and the dogged patience of listening to the author's story for the thousandth time with interest.

Writers have big, sensitive egos. As a first time author of a book, I had no clue that it would take me five years. About three years into the writing, I realized that I risked delaying publication unless I asked for help. Being protective about my work made asking for help difficult, but I'm glad that I asked. Sabra's willingness to work anywhere, whether on my living room couch or alongside me with a laptop in the cancer center infusion room were amazing personal sacrifices that she made for the sake of the book and which re-inspired me many times, especially when chemo wore me down.

In sometimes eighteen-hour working sessions where the intersection of determination, instinct, and a caffeine-soaked brain squeezed for the next great adjective collided, Sabra and I exacted phrases and worked our way through webbed topics sometimes too difficult for words. As for dedication, from now on I will visualize it in the following way: Sabra taking only her dog, Mocha and a copy of my unfinished book manuscript into an interior bathroom of her Dallas apartment as she hunkered down for the approach of a possible tornado. I am grateful to Sabra for her two years given to the publication of this book, for her many talents, honest feedback and needed criticisms for which I whole heartedly welcomed and respected.

When other publishers created havoc, sent me scads of rejection letters, or some not at all, and generally spun my head around into mush, Sabra kept cool and had reliable logic, at least on the outside. In the end, and because writers have big egos, I stayed true to my story. I refused to listen to the Park Avenue media machine that wanted my story told their way. They said that one more book about cancer was one too many. Through it all Sabra believed in my story. I am grateful for her willingness to learn, share, and come along for the ride when I wasn't sure when or where the book journey would end, or whether I'd live to finish writing it. Communication, trust and an endearing friendship have come from making this book, thanks to Sabra.

The publication of this book has been made possible with generous sponsorship from:

Harley Davidson of Dallas/Allen

And

Timberwolf Press

A Note To The Reader:

Always consult your physician before making health decisions, especially if you are being treated for cancer. Talk with your doctor, a nurse, social worker, clergy, family, a friend, or a support group if you are experiencing anxiety, or depression about cancer.

The opinions, viewpoints, and experiences shared in this book are not meant to diagnose, dissuade, or change cancer treatment plans. Each person's cancer journey is unique. Cancer types, methods of treatment, experiences and coping strategies are also unique to each person. The goal of the author is to provide education, offer insight and hope.

Permission has been obtained whether written or oral for the cancer story accounts and interviews in this book that are not those of the author.

The cancer prevention and awareness information found at the end of this book has been researched from numerous sources including: The Centers For Disease Control and Prevention, The American Cancer Society, The National Health Institute, The American Institute for Cancer Research, the National Cancer Institute, the Skin Cancer Foundation and numerous other sources. It is important to also note that information about cancer prevention, risk factors, causes and treatments are subject to change as new discoveries are made.

He who saves one life, it is as though he has saved the world.

—*Talmud*

**In Memory
Of
My Friends:**

Grace M. Strong and Maureen McVeigh-Carey

Dedication

Since the beginning of my cancer journey, several babies have been born among my family and friends. I have often lovingly referred to them as "Our Foundation Babies" and it is to them that I dedicate this book. With each new life there are newer possibilities. May we find a cure in your generation.

Michael Miller, Jr.
Joseph Miller
Hannah Riley Hartsfield
Kaitlyn Vess
Olivia Belle Osmond
Jake Osmond
Grant Michael Plumer
Reid Anthony Plumer
Jackson Cole Smithwick
Anna Cutic Mraovic

CONTENTS

Foreword

By Anna deHaro

Communications Director of Public Affairs for Clear Channel Radio

My father died of cancer when I was eighteen years old. I'd just started my freshman year in college and since I was the daughter of a professor, it meant a lot. My father's death came as no surprise, though it was as senseless as any accident. You see, my dad battled cancer for three years. Three years of hospital stays, chemotherapy, radiation, and prayers could not cure him, and though it feels strange to say it, his death was a relief. As my dad fought the injustice of this unstoppable monster, my family and I could do little else but love him, support him, and watch him be taken away.

Years earlier, the word cancer meant my astrological sign. "What's your sign?" people asked me and I'd say, "Cancer - Cancer the Crab to be exact." And boy, am I ever! Pick up any book about astrology signs and you'll find that those born under the sign of the Cancer Crab are known to be family-oriented, tenacious, and notoriously moody and sensitive. Check, check, check, and quadruple check. I fit the bill on all counts and when I was younger, I was actually quite proud of being a Cancerian, but in my freshman year of high school, the word Cancer took on a whole new meaning for me.

Everything changed one February evening. We were one of those families that always had dinner together. My father sat at the head of the table, my mother and I on either side, and where my brothers sat depended upon whether or not they were in an argument. One evening my parents said that we needed to have a family meeting and after dinner they gathered my two older brothers and me in the family room and told us that my father had cancer. cancer cancer Cancer CANCER….That ferocious word echoed in my head and all of a sudden cancer was no longer a harmless crab that symbolized my astrology sign. Cancer was the enemy. I remember sitting in our very green family room, with the green sofa and the green rug and the print that my mother bought at a garage sale with a woman that sat in a very green garden and I just let the horrible news sink in.

"Are you going to die?" my oldest brother asked my father.

"No," my father replied, "I have every intention of beating this disease, but I'm going to need your help. I'll need you guys to help your mother while I'm in the hospital."

Hospital? My father was never sick and now he talked about going into the hospital. How could this be? What did it mean? I'd soon find out.

For three years while my father was in and out of hospitals, my brothers and I traveled from family member to family member, and my mother focused all her attention on caring for my dad. From that moment on, cancer was a member of our household. We didn't set a place for it at the dinner table but it was there. My parents' bedroom looked like a hospital suite. Medicines filled the top of the nightstand, along with little plastic syringes and water pitchers with plastic cups that were probably remnants from a previous hospital stay. I'd walk into my parents' room, pray that my father would be okay, and as he slept, I'd check to make sure he still breathed. It's been years since my dad's illness, but I remember it all so well.

Not a day goes by that I don't think about him and wish that he were still alive. Why couldn't my dad be one of the lucky ones that I've heard speak at cancer events as their family looks on with pride? Don't get me wrong. I'm very proud of my father. He fought a valiant fight and it wasn't until much later that I realized how tough he really was. My dad never complained as he battled cancer and he actually made cancer treatments look easy because he didn't want his children to see how scared he was. At the time, I didn't know how difficult chemotherapy really was, but a food-poisoning incident helped me to understand it better.

About a month before my father died, I visited family in Monterrey, Mexico, and one evening we went to a seafood restaurant for dinner. A short time later, I was so sick that my aunt found me passed out on the bathroom floor. I was rushed to a nearby hospital where doctors thought that appendicitis was the cause of my illness and wanted to operate. In my weakened state, I begged my aunt not to let them cut me open and it's a good thing because I had food poisoning.

I've never felt so awful. I was nauseous for weeks and the mere sight of food made my stomach turn. When I was finally able to go back home to South Texas I told my father about my experience and he told me that's what chemotherapy felt like for him. He was so calm when he said it, as if the experience was as ordinary as a spring rain. At that moment, the reality of cancer treatments hit me like a bomb.

Finally, he pulled the curtain back to let me know what it was like to battle cancer. On so many occasions, I went to the cancer center with my father for his treatments and he never hinted to me that it affected him in the way that he revealed. My father's story is not unlike the millions of other fathers, mothers, sisters, brothers, aunts, uncles, wives, or husbands who have fought the mighty "C" word. Naively, I thought that a cure would be found for this insidious disease a couple years after my father's death, but here we are, so many years later, and the battle rages on across the globe. That's where Michelle Miller comes in.

I first met Michelle in 2003 through my position as director of Public Affairs at a Dallas radio station. One day, I received an email about a woman in nearby Allen, Texas, who not only battled cancer, but was also building a cancer monument dedicated to all who had battled cancer, and those who still battled. This monument was unlike any other and would honor the courage of those who fought; it would show the world that we wouldn't forget, nor give up in the effort to find a cure for cancer. I was awestruck and compelled to hear more so I e-mailed Michelle and set up an interview for our Sunday morning Public Affairs Show. I wanted to honor my father and all the others who've gone toe-to-toe with cancer. I wanted to help build the monument. Once I learned all about The Cancer Monument, I was convinced that the time had arrived for it and it would be built. I still get chills when I think about how Michelle, in the midst of her own cancer battle, envisioned The Cancer Monument, but that's her story to tell and you're about to read all about it.

When I first heard about the Cancer Monument, it made perfect sense and I wondered why it hadn't been done before. The public need for such a monument has always been present. Cancer has taken so many of our loved ones. Cancer is the number one killer of Americans and a worldwide epidemic with no cure. Why hadn't anyone else loudly proclaimed that those who battle in the "War on Cancer" are heroes? The answer is simple. It was always Michelle's role to lead us all to The Cancer Monument, as though it waited for her. Michelle's drive and passion compels people to get involved and there is no one else who can convey this powerful, worldwide message so well because she lives it.

Over the years, I've met many people who've lost a loved one to cancer. Whether a parent, a child, or a friend, one thing that I know to be true is that we all love to talk about our loved ones who've fought cancer with valor. They are our Heroes. It's as if by talking about them, we keep them alive A retold story shared with others has the power to transport us back to that moment in time: we see their face, hear their laughter, remember conversations, and for that second they are in the room with us again. I used to fantasize that if I won the lotto, I'd have a building at the University of Texas Pan American in South Texas named after my father, or maybe one at Southern Methodist University in Dallas.

My father got his law degree from SMU and I thought it would be a nice way to immortalize and honor him there. But those kinds of honors usually go to people who are famous and rich like politicians, big time celebrities, philanthropists, or people who win the lotto and can afford to buy a university building. I wanted the world to know my dad. I fantasized that one day someone would ask how the "Rafael de Haro Law Library" got its name, and then my father's story would be told. They'd know about the man that was not only my dad, but a man who loved the law and believed that to teach law was a much greater reward than to practice it. Granted, the law library is just a silly fantasy but when I share the story with friends who have suffered through the loss of a parent, they always confess to share the same sort of fantasy and perhaps that is why The Cancer Monument strikes a chord with so many people.

The Cancer Monument is the people's monument and will accomplish so many things on our behalf. It will honor the soldiers in the War on Cancer; help to heal the grief stricken, and will be a legacy of prevention, education, and research advocacy. We want people to know about our loved ones – our Heroes in The War on Cancer. We want a place where our voices can be heard. The Cancer Monument will be our place. I feel blessed to know that The Cancer Monument takes such an unconventional approach to the War on Cancer and that the end result will be visible, tangible and for you and me for generations to come. Michelle and everyone in her organization have tremendous love in their hearts for this monument and those whose lives it will touch. It is a comfort for me to know that such dedicated individuals are in the fight for us all. Michelle Miller inspires and humbles me because of her enthusiasm and optimism. Heck, I'm tired just as soon as I walk into my house and see a sink full of dirty dishes. But though Michelle has had to deal with her cancer for a while, through it all she remains focused on The Cancer Monument and reminds me of the battery commercial with the bunny who keeps on going. If you spend just a few minutes with Michelle, you too, will be caught up in the magic of this once-in-a-lifetime opportunity dedicated with love to our soldiers in the War on Cancer. There are many times in my life when I've believed that things happen for a reason. Some call that fate. The Cancer Monument is fate unveiled. The curtain is up now and it is offered to us all with loving hearts and hands. Now, it is the duty of each one of us to take the next step in this journey by inscribing the names of our loved ones who've battled cancer so that The Cancer Monument can be built.

Introduction

By Michelle Miller

Only two months into my cancer battle I was struck with the following thought: If cancer is a war, then those who fight the battle are soldiers. So, where is our monument?

This question, which changed my life forever, now brings hope and inspiration to thousands of people throughout the world. Our culture pays homage to unlikely sources of heroism. Arrogant athletes, drug-addicted, or even criminal music industry idols, daredevil adventurers who jump off cliffs, and privileged Hollywood movie stars are those whom we gladly celebrate. My story isn't about any of those people. I'm an ordinary person and I'm a cancer survivor. However, my cancer story has an uncommon twist, different than most, and may even have the potential to change your life too. As a result of my cancer diagnosis, I now celebrate and honor the type of hero that you probably don't think about in the ordinary course of every day—the Heroes in the War on Cancer. In May of 2000, fate met with circumstance and The Cancer Monument was born. As a result, I now lead The Cancer Monument, Incorporated; a non-profit charity. This compelling, national campaign effort is gathering 60,000 Honoree names to be inscribed on the monument's black, granite walls. To date, people from 20 states have submitted names of those who have battled cancer. As you read my story, ask yourself: Who is my Hero in The War on Cancer?

I've taken an unexpected cancer journey and yet, I feel that it was a destined one, mostly for the purpose of building Cancer Monument, but though The Cancer Monument began with me, it is by no means a one-woman show. Legions of talented, truly remarkable people have joined me in the quest and each one deserves high praise for their commitment to this unique mission. The Cancer Monument story has never been told before as it is here in this true account. However, you will only read about the first 5 years because it is a story that has not yet ended. The ending is up to each of you. With your help, I anticipate the day, very soon, when we'll all stand together to rejoice in a monument built by love, faith, and a commitment to a great cause.

On the monument's behalf, these past few years have brought us all hard work in the form of sweat, negotiation, and the type of worry, tears, and unimaginable love known only to parents for their child. As a result of such dedication, we are on the way to The Cancer Monument. It is now possible to have this first-ever, legacy structure and your part, as a concerned citizen, is to inscribe the name, or names of your Honored Heroes. In doing so, you will help build this incredible monument that will stand tall and proud for generations.

By now, you are probably asking - How did The Cancer Monument begin? Well, it began with my basic and primal need to cope with cancer. The matter of coping was and still is the hardest part of my cancer journey and is the central purpose of this book. Throughout my story, my need to cope yields uncommon forms, like The Cancer Monument, never imagined, or made possible before by anyone's cancer journey. Until there is a cure, cancer is with us and lurks in the shadows for its next prey: a child, a mother, a son, or a friend. Whatever your cancer type or disease stage, whether you are a caregiver, or a friend of someone who has cancer, we all have to cope with cancer, like it or not. Many will gladly give advice on how they've coped with cancer but what works for some, will not necessarily work for others. Education is our answer to a better life in the midst of cancer and the best way to learn new ideas is to be open-minded and involved in the process.

Coping is hard work and is often a matter overlooked until we are deep in crisis. Like a force from a tsunami wave, once I was diagnosed with cancer, every reality and belief system I owned was quickly pounded, pummeled, and drowned. Learning how to cope became my first major survival challenge and required honest self-reflection, creativity, and tremendous flexibility in an uncharted state of crisis. I didn't want to be categorized as a victim of cancer, nor did I merely want to exist with cancer. I wanted to thrive! But, how do you cope with an encroaching cancerous enemy when there are no rulebooks or road maps to ensure your success? I fought back by first disabling my enemy's manifesto of despair with my stronger will to live. In doing so, I maintained a positive outlook that set into motion a pattern of enlightenment, which enabled me to perceive the War on Cancer differently than most. Being involved in the pursuit of life left me fewer moments to obsess about my death, and soon I became empowered by adversity.

Thinking like a soldier was one of my major coping strategies and was a stepping-stone in my thought process on the way to The Cancer Monument. Frequently, I'd visualize myself in full combat gear, muddied but strong, I'd hurl imaginary grenades and exchange hellish dialogues against enemy forces. When the grenades were used up, I'd engage in brutal hand-to-hand combat to gain back territory long since taken within me by a malicious infiltrator. On one particular day, in one incredible moment of life-altering clarity, I envisioned The Cancer

Monument. The journey began long before my diagnosis.

Wars are never won with just a single weapon. The same is true for the War on Cancer. Like artillery, The Cancer Monument is part of the solution. Though it is not yet built, it does the job it is intended to do as we campaign throughout the nation to build it. The monument raises awareness, which may help to prevent new cancers, and provides thousands of people with peace, hope, inspiration, and a hallowed ground of their own in which to give thanks, to be honored, remembered, and celebrated for valor and courage under fire. The Cancer Monument offers to us all the rightful and unique perspective of what it means to battle and cope with cancer. Public knowledge of the monument has lifted despair from lonely, frightened faces and brought hope to the heavy hearts of the grief-stricken. I've witnessed entire rooms of people, men and women alike, burst into tears of joy to know that such a structure waits for them and is intended to honor them or their loved ones who've battled in the War on Cancer. I've witnessed families, businesses, and boardrooms, local governments, churches, other cancer organizations, schools, and entire communities across several states, come together in support of this monument. The message is the same; "Thank you, finally, a monument for us!"

The time has come for The Cancer Monument. It is now possible and is the new definition and positive, visual perception of the War on Cancer. The Cancer Monument is the people's monument and will be built for the people and by the people. It will educate, inspire, and most importantly, will allow millions who've been affected by cancer to emerge from the cloak of shame, despair, and the cultural grip of a powerful stigma of victimization. The Cancer Monument replaces negativity with new hope, courage, and purpose gained from the more assertive philosophy that the diagnosed are soldier-heroes in a declared War on Cancer. I've never negotiated with the cancer enemy and will never raise the white flag of defeat. The Cancer Monument is my mantra, building it is my torch of progress, and endures as my driving purpose to get out of bed every day, lock horns with cancer, and make a difference in the world too.

My own need to cope with cancer collided with the unmet need in others to have a cancer monument and represents a small part of a timeless human story. Oddly enough, within seconds after receiving my cancer diagnosis, I knew that I'd write a book and immediately began a cancer journal. My cancer journal has evolved to become this book. As I wrote my thoughts and feelings, I unknowingly recorded my own coping mechanisms and my transformational journey to build The Cancer Monument. Along the way, I've come to know the many stories of our Cancer Monument Heroes. Through their family and friends the legacy of these incredible people live on to teach us hope, courage, and love. A few of their stories are shared in this book. My ultimate goal for you as my reader is to fill your lungs to capacity with re-born inspiration, to brighten your spirit, maybe even to laugh a little, and nurture your mind with fresh ammunition so that newer perspectives on coping with cancer may be yours.

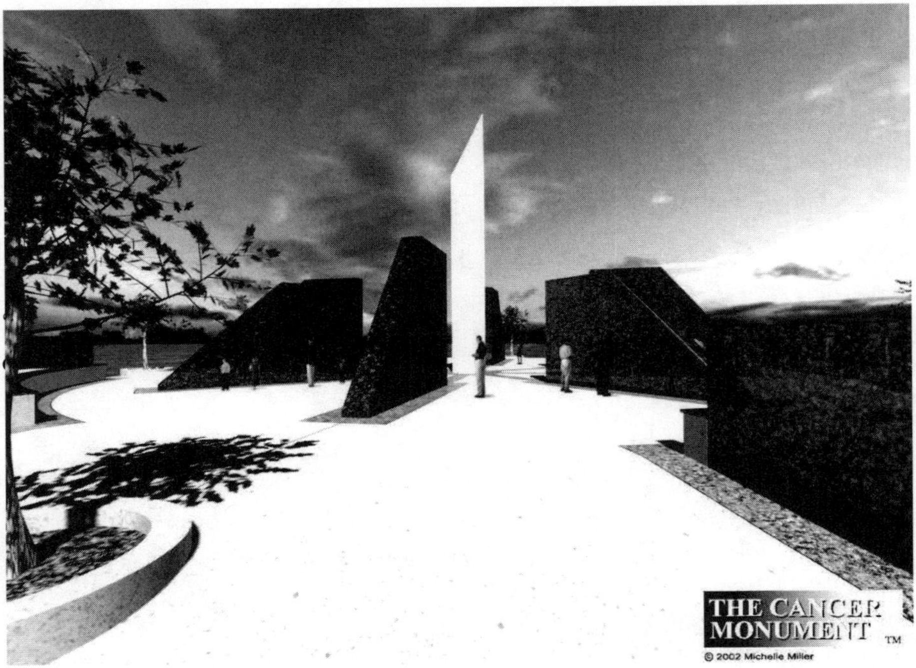

"The human mind, once stretched to a new idea, never goes back to its original dimensions."

— Oliver Holmes

Chapter 1
On The Battleground

"So this is the War on Cancer," I thought.

The nurse pointed to the chemo bags that hung above me and explained what would happen next, "This one is called 'Red Devil'; It's the fourth drug in your chemo cocktail." This potent combination of liquids didn't include a cabana and poolside waiter. There'd be no plump, red cherries, exotic flavors, or pink paper umbrellas, although pain and disbelief were on tap. Joey and I looked at each other. The reality was clear. I had cancer. We didn't know it then, but four years later, we'd still be in the fight.

I watched the chemo poison drip down an IV tube and into a surgically implanted medi-port in my chest. Joey, my husband of just a few weeks, sat nearby and worked from his laptop, and cell phone. A part of me still hoped that a mistake had been made. Every time I was stuck with a fresh needle I wanted to scream out, "Are you all crazy? I'm not sick!" We were supposed to be on our honeymoon in Jamaica, not in a cancer center. I tried to relax and thought back on the sequence of events that brought me there. Just a few weeks earlier, a seamstress made final alterations to my wedding dress and I gave more concern to my waistline than to a raised lymph node discovered by my doctor during a routine physical.

"It might be a fat deposit, I've seen this type of thing before," my doctor said on that pivotal day, "but let's play it safe and have it checked right away." But, there I was, at my first chemo treatment and wished that a little extra fat was what ailed me instead of the cancer tumor that resided in my chest. How could I possibly have cancer when my life was just beginning, I wondered. My mind scrambled to make logic from chaos, but was suddenly distracted by another concern. I couldn't breathe. Gray puffs of smoke exited my nose. I coughed out my words to the nurse, "Excuse me, but can you slow down the chemo a bit? I think my nostril hairs are on fire."

***

My original call to Dr. Bannister in late March 2000 was due to a pulled lower back muscle caused by months of aggressive workouts. The strained area throbbed with every movement and periodically triggered unexpected shards of pain that caused me to wince and arch in agony, which was especially embarrassing at work. I was overdue for a physical anyway and figured that since I'd soon be married and planned to start a family, a doctor's visit was in order. Somewhere between conference calls and a myriad of wedding-related appointments, I managed to squeeze in an exam during a work lunch hour.

As the doctor went through the exam, I chatted about my wedding in Jamaica, only two months and eighteen days away. Suddenly, a pronounced crease of concern appeared on Dr. Bannister's forehead as she pressed and kneaded on my collarbone area. What could be wrong with my collarbone when I was there for a strained back muscle I wondered?

"Have you had any recent night sweats, itchy skin, unexplained fevers, or rapid weight loss?" she asked me.

"Not at all," I said. "I feel fabulous except for my back," and pointed as if to remind her why I was there in the first place. But my pulled back muscle wasn't anything more serious than what a few days' rest and some anti-inflammatory pills couldn't fix. The doctor had a much greater concern. Dr. Bannister grew quiet and continued to examine my neck and collarbone area before giving a weighted exhale that contained this memorable question;

"Have you ever noticed this lump in your neck?"

"Excuse me?" I retorted. "I don't have a lump in my neck." My New York accent couldn't be restrained. I figured if there was a lump, I would've known about it.

"Here," my doctor said, "feel that," and pressed my fingers against a swollen lymph node in my right clavicle. "Let's not be alarmed just yet," she said as she wrote orders for an immediate CAT scan and X-ray. "I'd feel much better if you'd have this checked out right now," she said. "I don't want you to go back to work until you do."

I didn't have time for unplanned events and didn't want to be inconvenienced by the likelihood of several more hours at the hospital for nothing. Though I was full of impatience, I wasn't about to dismiss the doctor's orders. I did as she instructed and never once imagined that a cancer diagnosis awaited me. Why in the world would I think that I had cancer anyway? I was thirty-three years old, athletic, hadn't had a cold or so much as taken an aspirin in over a year. Some even considered me a bit of a health "nut." I was almost militaristic in my approach to good health and exercised six days a week at the gym, sometimes twice a day, and had a home gym on top of that. I drank at least two liters of water daily and simultaneously curled an 8-pound weight while on the phone.

Despite it all, the test results given to me on April 1st were no joke. Joey and I returned to Dr. Bannister's office for results of the X-ray, CT, and biopsy. As we entered the tiny exam room, the scan images hung one by one on a lit display board. Though I wasn't an expert in human anatomy, I'd taken a fair amount of biology in college and knew what a normal human body should look like.

"Wow," I said, "whose scans are those?" and pointed to a round mass in the sternum situated between the lungs "What's that strange round thing in the center? It's not a heart."

"No," said Dr. Bannister. Her voice shook at the prospect of giving bad news. "It's not a heart at all. It's a mass, about the size of a large orange, and those are your scans."

My knees went weak and I sat down.

"I'm so sorry to have to tell you that you have cancer. Hodgkin's Lymphoma, to be exact," she said.

Joey and I remained calm but with each utterance of the word "cancer," the tiny exam room tightened its grip. The tearful approach was too predictable, so I resisted. It simply would've amounted to wasted energy and no resolution. At that point, none of it was logical and I couldn't cry, nor be mad, or even scared. How could I possibly have cancer when I didn't feel sick, I questioned. The most serious medical conditions I'd ever experienced were a tonsillectomy, a few root canals, and impacted wisdom teeth. I figured someone had fouled up at the lab and this little miscommunication would be straightened out in a few days, along with an apology, and good-natured laughter. As Dr. Bannister continued to talk about success rates and treatment options for Hodgkins' Lymphoma, memories of my friend Maureen barreled their way to the forefront of my mind. We had more in common than she'd ever know. Shortly after giving birth to her only child, a cancerous tumor was discovered wrapped around her heart. Maureen fought cancer like a true soldier and her courage and hope were an awesome sight to witness. She died just before I moved to Texas in the spring of

1998.

Think. You've got to think through this, I thought. I glanced at Joey seated next to me; his legs were comfortably crossed and with his usual air of calm he took notes into his Palm Pilot organizer as Dr. Bannister spoke. My goodness, I thought, doesn't anything rattle this man? Since Joey was in control, I could escape from the moment, if only for a few seconds to collect my thoughts. As I went to a place in my mind, unreachable to anyone, the words that filled the room whooshed in my ears like the sounds in a seashell. My mind flashed: our wedding…the promotion at work…and graduate school. What would happen to my life now? A strangely out-of-place word re-focused my attention: Lucky.

"You sure are lucky this was caught early and before you started to display symptoms," Dr. Bannister remarked. I didn't feel lucky at all. I had cancer. Dr. Bannister rose from her chair, hugged us both, and handed me a business card that read: Dr. Smith, Oncologist.

"Make an appointment with him right away," she said and gave me one last hug before Joey and I marched forward to meet with our destiny. As we drove home, we reviewed our previous hour with Dr. Bannister.

"Joey, do you think it's true?" I asked. "Do you think I really have cancer?"

"Well, it seems so after everything we just heard," he said with caution. "Let's meet with this oncologist and see what he says." Joey finished. I stared at the doctor's business card.

"On-col-o-gy," I said the word out loud. I had a good vocabulary, but was unfamiliar with that word. I tried to remember root words from my many years of study in Italian, Greek, Hebrew, and Spanish. Ology - the study of - I knew what that part meant, but the study of what I wondered. Onc. What did that part mean? Ignorance, innocence, and denial volleyed.

"What's an oncologist?" I asked Joey

"A cancer doctor," he said.

"Oh," I said. Suddenly, the thought of being a cancer patient made me feel like a shackled prisoner at the mercy of fate and science. A tumor resided in my chest and for all I knew, it might cause me to combust at any moment as we careened down the expressway. Clear the area! Run! Run! I screamed in my head. I wanted to protect Joey too but didn't know how. The thought of cancer made me want to escape, run for cover, or find the nearest alien space ship. If only somehow I could leave my diseased body behind - anything - anything to just get away from the horrible doom that I was sure awaited me. "You can't run, you have to fight," I told myself. My thoughts turned again to Joey. He didn't sign up for cancer. He deserved to have a life as he imagined.

"Joey," I said, "Let's be practical about this. The rules have changed. So, under the circumstances, you don't have to marry me."

"What are you talking about?" he said in astonishment. "I'll turn this car around right now and find the nearest Justice of the Peace." He wasn't calm anymore. "I'll marry you this minute if that's what you want."

"Well, I'd prefer a religious ceremony like we planned," I said. "But, how can I marry you when I don't know my future? You deserve to have the kind of life that you want."

"Nobody knows the future when they get married and it shouldn't matter, if you love the person," he said.

"But we're not married yet," I reminded him. "I don't have a choice, but you do. This is my problem, why make it yours? You can walk away right now and save yourself a lot of heartache. I'd never hold it against you if you did and will love you just the same," I said.

"I don't want to walk away. I want to fight this with you. We're a team," Joey said.

"All I can promise you right now is that I love you." I said.

"Well, that's good enough for me! In sickness and in health, till death do us part," Joey reminded. "What do you think those wedding vows mean? Do you think I take my commitments lightly?" He seemed insulted at the very idea.

"No," I said, "but many people do when tragedy strikes,"

"Well, I'm not one of those people. I've felt those wedding vows in my heart since the day I asked you to move to Texas with me. Our wedding day doesn't make those vows true. We do. It's you and me babe, all the way." Ordinarily, Joey is a man of few words, but that day, he had a lot to say. A tremendous sense of responsibility was lifted from my shoulders. I didn't want him to feel obligated by our engagement if he had any second thoughts, or worse, marry me out of pity. I wanted to assure Joey that he still had an option. So, like a bird that's free to fly away from danger, I released him, and was grateful to know that even cancer wouldn't make him flee.

"So what's it going to be? Are you skipping out on me now, or what?" Joey insisted.

"No way," I said. "But a Jamaican wedding doesn't seem practical at this point. Let's have a ceremony in Dallas instead," I said. Joey smiled.

"Fine by me," he said, "whatever you want."

"And one more thing," I said. "Can we move up the wedding date? I don't want to be a bald bride."

As soon as we got home I made an appointment with the oncologist.

"Two weeks? I can't wait that long," I said, "this is an emergency. I have cancer!" The receptionist understood my alarm. I took the appointment anyway and learned soon enough that all patients at this doctor's office had the same emergency as me - cancer. Once handed a cancer diagnosis, there was too much to do with survival being a top priority. I groaned as I made a list of about fifty people to call with the news. Family members, friends, co-workers, and professors all needed to be made aware of my cancer and the wedding plan changes. From many, I anticipated waves of insurmountable tears and wild hysteria, and wanted no part of any sad spectacle in which I'd be the star attraction. I just wanted to stay level-headed, focused, and didn't want to be sucked into a tide of unanswerable questions. I wanted to survive. Everyone, including me, would want to know why, how, and the next step. What was the prognosis? When would a treatment plan begin and for how long? Some answers I'd never know for sure, but a great deal of information was yet to be learned from the oncologist. Joey and I sat in our living room and began the reorganization of our lives.

"Okay," I said, "how do we want to play this? Let's get a game plan."

"Well, we can't change who we are," Joey said, "so let's handle things the way we always do. We'll fact-find and then make a logical, educated decision based on evidence." Joey's reliable calm was the perfect antidote to chaos and he'd keep me grounded even when things went from bad to worse.

"I agree," I said. "I think it's important that we maintain a normal routine as best as possible. We'll live our lives around cancer. That's our policy," I said.

"We'll just deal with situations as they come up," Joey finished.

"Okay, now what about other people? We're about to be bombarded with a hundred opinions and emotions." I envisioned the likely scenarios and my chest tightened in anticipation. "I'll need to keep a level head and stay positive," I insisted, "and I won't be around negative people."

"Well, people are only human. They'll cry and have all kinds of reactions," Joey said. "There's nothing you can do about that. It's only natural to be sad about sad news, but their views and sentiments don't have any impact on our lives unless we allow it. You're in control," Joey said. "They'll take your emotional cue. Just let people know where you stand." It was one thing to make family and friends understand my needs; that seemed easy enough. But, I also knew that because I now had cancer, society in general viewed me as a victim and the negative force from that collective viewpoint already made me feel unsupported and angry.

I remembered years earlier, I'd heard a second-hand story about someone who'd returned to work after a battle with cancer. To my disbelief, her co-workers were actually concerned about catching cancer so whenever the cancer survivor left her desk, they'd spray and disinfect her workspace. I also remembered another story about a holiday party that a few wouldn't attend because one of the guests was on chemotherapy and they thought that their own health would somehow be affected by her presence. I knew both of these stories to be ignorant and cruel from the moment I heard them. Cancer is not contagious. But cancer was now my reality, and based on history, I couldn't deny that some people could be downright dense. I didn't want to deal with it. I just wanted to get through my ordeal, be healthy again, and live my life. Yet, in the minds of many, I was beaten before I'd even begun to fight. The truth was, either I wouldn't be beaten at all, or I'd go down in a glorious knockdown, drag-out fight to the death. A victim? No way. Though I'd have to fight in order to win my body back from cancer's grip, my character, my soul, myself - those were mine and couldn't be touched by any disease. I'd use them as weapons when cancer drugs, research, and insurance companies failed to help, but the everyday struggle of coping remained my burden. In the battle ahead, I'd have my fair share of sadness and tears, but early in my cancer battle, it was my good fortune to be quickly reacquainted with the power within myself. With that emerged an enormous turning point; my defense plan for the War on Cancer was underway.

Strategy equaled safety for me and without it I felt vulnerable. The next two weeks dragged on and along the way, the lack of information about my treatment plan and prognosis conjured up and festered new and old fears. Would I be harassed out of my job, or dropped by my health insurance? Would doctors be compassionate or hold me responsible for my illness? More importantly, would medical professionals have the desire or ability to fight for my recovery? The idea of placing my life into the hands of strangers fanned a forest fire of insecurities for me. I needed to feel confident about a medical plan of action and urgently needed to begin a relationship of trust with an oncologist. I called the oncologist's office again and at the sound of the receptionist's voice, my composure was lost for a few seconds as I sobbed half-intelligible questions about the doctor's credentials, character, and bedside manner. The receptionist pieced my words together and assured me that I'd be in good hands, and told me she'd send some literature in the mail for me. A few days later, the information packet arrived and I poured over every word, checked sources, and was impressed. The definition of oncology was now clear.

***

Joey and I were married on April 16, 2000, and not only did I have hair but it looked great too. We were so proud that day as we exchanged our vows before God and knew that we'd already passed a great test. Our friends David and Carolyn were our witnesses and there was barely a dry eye in the room. Family members from New York and Indiana flew in to Dallas to celebrate our joyful day. After the ceremony we went to a lovely reception that our friends organized. The cake was beautiful, the food was fantastic and the champagne flowed. Music and laughter filled the room as the photographer captured the special moments of the day. Thoughts of cancer were far in the background until at one point during the reception, an out-of-town guest took me aside and asked, 'whether I thought that it was a good idea to rush into marriage since I now had cancer,' that perhaps, 'we should've waited until I was cured.' If it were proper or legal for a bride to punch a guest in the face, I would've done so right then and there. I was shocked and insulted by her remarks. I signaled Joey over and insisted that she repeat what she said. Her eyes grew wide at being put on the spot as she clutched her husband's arm for support. The poor man didn't talk much and hadn't had his own opinion in more than thirty years. With tone and tempers in check, we let her know that her sentiments were inappropriate and unwelcome. We'd been engaged for a year and a half and were to be married only weeks before my diagnosis. We were adults who'd made a decision together, and most importantly, we loved each other.

"Isn't love the reason why people marry?" Joey inquired.

"I suppose so," she said with a vacant stare. She could no longer defend her verbal spew. Joey and I continued our celebration despite her efforts to stomp on our joy. I had assumed that cancer would be the uninvited party crasher but was shocked to discover that a traitor existed among the invited.

After the reception, we continued our celebration with family at one of our favorite sushi restaurants. To this day, the restaurant staff still remembers Joey and me as "the wedding party." Our wedding day turned out the way fate intended and was more beautiful, and more memorable than any carefully orchestrated event could offer. But, I have to admit that from time to time, the loss of our Jamaican wedding paradise stings my pride and makes me a little sad for what might have been. Whenever those thoughts creep in to rob me of my joy, I remind myself that I already have the greatest reward: I am married to the man I love and I am alive. As for our wedding guest who thought I was rushing into marriage, her husband was diagnosed with cancer two years later.

Finally, the appointment day with the oncologist arrived. Dr. Smith explained that Hodgkin's Lymphoma is an immune system cancer, a part of the lymphatic system which runs like a highway throughout the body. Because of this, surgical removal of the tumor in my chest could likely spread cancer to unaffected areas and was not an option. He continued to explain that Hodgkin's Lymphoma occurs in about one percent of all cancer cases and is considered the most curable of all cancer types. I was prescribed a standard treatment protocol of four to six months of chemotherapy intended to shrink the tumor, followed by a minimum of four to six weeks of targeted radiation to the tumor site, to kill any remaining cancer cells.

"Is there any way that the test results could be wrong?" Joey questioned.

"No, the tests are conclusive," said the doctor. Dr. Smith also said that because of the slow growth rate of my cancer type, the tumor might have taken ten years or more to get to the size of an orange. Then, he explained the fortune of my diagnosis, "Consider yourself very lucky, since without symptoms there'd be no need for a doctor to order tests and your tumor would not have been detected for maybe another year or two."

He went on to describe a typical scenario of misdiagnosis. Patients with continuous fevers, rapid weight loss, or a relentless cough might be given medicines for common ailments like allergies or the flu. In the meantime, cancer would continue to grow into their organs, or worse, bone marrow. As an oncologist, Dr. Smith saw this type of desperate scenario all too often and sometimes, it was too late. But there were success stories too, lots of them, and Joey and I prayed that I'd live to see 2001.

I was in Stage 2 and a-symptomatic, which meant that I displayed no symptoms. The tumor was above my diaphragm, involved no organs, or bone marrow. Compared to other cancer patients I was lucky, Dr. Smith said. Dr. Bannister said that too, but it certainly didn't make me feel like a game show winner. I didn't feel lucky at all. I had cancer. But as a matter of perspective, I understood then that my situation could've been far worse and was for many others.

"Did I stand too close to the microwave?" I attempted to make my question sound humorous, but I was completely serious. "How did this happen, Dr. Smith? I don't fall into any of the risk groups."

"First of all, you did nothing wrong," he said. I was relieved to hear that much. "Science still doesn't know why some people get cancer and others don't, but we're learning all the time and have better medicines than ever before."

So, according to the standard treatment plan, I'd be free of cancer in about six months and back to a normal life. Dr. Smith was dedicated to the field of oncology, lymphoma research, and had an intriguing, cerebral humor that would help pull me back down to reality in times of stress. Most importantly, he was committed to my health. I no longer had any fears about oncologists and my prognosis for being cured was ninety percent or higher. Joey and I felt confident in the plan and were ready to wage War on Cancer. A few days later, the nurse read off a long list of chemotherapy side effects to Joey and me from the frayed pages of a thick manual to help prepare us for chemotherapy. We were distressed over some of them, which could include residual effects thirty years later like organ failure, secondary cancers, or even death. Survival required risks.

In exhaustive detail, the nurse discussed protocol and gave us an all too unbelievable synopsis of how our lives would be for the next several months. Nothing was negotiable. I'd have medicines to help prevent vomiting. I'd make weekly lab visits for blood draws and had to immediately call the doctor if there were convulsions, seizures, a fever of over a hundred degrees, rash, swelling, difficulty breathing, or urinating and the list continued. My eyes raced to Joey in desperation as the pages on chemotherapy side effects turned. I wondered if I was doing the right thing and if maybe, somehow, Joey could ease my burden. After all, Joey was the Director of Software Solutions for a medical billing company and for fifteen years, had made his professional career to provide long-range technical solutions. I needed a fast fix to this urgent problem.

As the nurse continued our patient education segment, Joey read the anxiety in my eyes. He leaned toward me, reached for my hand,

and his expression was clear. He couldn't fix this problem. My mind drifted as acceptance slowly washed over me. Unlike matters at work, or anywhere else, I wouldn't be able to bargain the terms of cancer. I was used to operating in a structured world. This problem offered little recourse. I couldn't send it back to the kitchen; get an upgrade, a refund, draft a proposal, picket, or write to my Congressman. This problem was mine and there were no laws in which to find safety.

The nurse continued to read off the list of cautions and dangers. My mind was far away as I mechanically nodded and scribbled my signature when prompted. Joey was fully in the moment and filled out a stack of medical forms as I attempted to mentally reorganize my entire life. I was startled back into reality with the statement: "Honey, it'll be about fifteen days before it all falls out." The nurse's mouth seemed to move in slow motion as she pointed to my hair. Joey put his arm around my shoulder and gave me a squeeze for reassurance.

"It'll grow back," he said.

The date of my first chemo fast approached. I entered this strange and frightening experience with a journal of blank pages thinking that writing would help me better cope. My first entry reads:

May 4, 2000 'A Trip To Hell'

My knees nearly buckled upon entering the chemo room. Am I going to die here? There are radioactive emblems posted everywhere. Everyone seems friendly. I hear no painful screams, or sights of terror and anarchy. I see no devils, pitchforks, pointy horns, witch's cauldrons, or flames. What do my eyes see in the corner of the room? In a large wicker basket sits a mound of cookies and chocolate bars. If hell is serving up chocolate, maybe this won't be so bad after all! Somehow, I still don't think that I belong here. How can I have cancer when I don't feel sick? Today is the first day of chemotherapy. I am writing in my journal as the nurse hooks up the four drugs called a 'cocktail' to an I.V. tube. I had asked for Margaritas on ice, but it wasn't the cocktail they had in mind for me. The I.V. is plugged into the port in my chest, which was implanted into a vein this morning at 7 o'clock. I'm supposed to be in Jamaica right now, lounging at the pool, dancing, and walking the beach by moonlight with Joey. I'm getting chemo instead. I've decided to make the best of it.

***

Later that evening, I lay on the couch and grabbed my chest in pain. I struggled for breath. Joey was on the other side of the house and with the strength of a deflated balloon, I squeaked out his name for help. Once he was alongside me, I whispered, "Quick. Call the doctor. I can't get enough air in my lungs. I don't think this is normal."

I was no longer in a normal land. I was on the battlegrounds of cancer. After being admitted to the hospital, x-rays revealed a tiny puncture in my lung, which happened during the medi-port surgery that morning. I was put on oxygen and the lung healed within a couple of days. I had to make a conscious decision to try and live around my crisis yet I was angered at the injustice of it all. I now had to deal with one more obstacle thrown in my path. Couldn't anyone help lighten my load just a little? But I was only at the beginning of a long battle filled with frustration. Over the next couple of years, somewhere between the grenades and rocket launchers, science and I teamed up on many battlegrounds in order to liberate me from cancer. When we lost, I was left to pick up the pieces and find a way to cope through still more cancer. I was consistently baffled and frustrated about why science didn't know more after billions of dollars had been spent on research. Was research money mishandled? Were people asleep at the microscope? Did anyone really care? I was worried that I might drop dead before science found a cure. Many people had, including my friend Maureen. I refused to place all trust in the propaganda machine, which dictates that research is the only hope. Research was a big part of the equation, but I wasn't so convinced that it was my only hope. Maybe hope existed in other forms. I was willing to explore the options and make new ones too in order to save my life.

The hope that I'd keep my hair didn't last. On the fifteenth day after my first chemotherapy treatment, a follicular coup began with a tingly sensation on my scalp, just as the nurses predicted. For days, chunks of hair silently fell out on my pillow, the floor, plates of food, and anywhere else I stayed for too long. Weeks earlier, the oncologist and nurses explained that chemotherapy kills rapidly growing cells like skin, nails, the lining of the digestive tract, cancer cells, and also, hair.

But no one explained to me how devastated and lost I'd feel, or how I'd cope through it all. With my hair falling out in gobs all over the house, denial, even just a little, was not an option any longer. The loss of my hair was the most visual symbol of my illness and seemed even more traumatic than the prospect of death. My hair was an extension of my femininity and was more like a limb than just hair. If the loss of my hair was the external view of chemo's effects, I wondered what other cellular wars took place on the inside of my body. As gobs of hair fell from my head, I felt wedged between two battling forces: chemotherapy that was supposed to save me but could also kill me, and the stealth of a cancer enemy who abided by no treaty, or ethics.

Alone in the bathroom, I stood in front of the mirror and mourned over the reflection before me. I was nearly bald, bruised from weeks of needles, scarred with bright red surgery incisions, and bloated. I didn't recognize my own reflection and with that realization, I felt pangs of terror. If I didn't recognize my reflection, I wondered if I existed at all. Suddenly, I was seized with the thought that I might fade into nothingness and be dead and buried before my thirty-fifth birthday.

"Where are you, Michelle?" I said to my reflection and the fact that my mouth moved told me that it was definitely me in the mirror. I was scared and didn't know what to do next. "You're inside," I answered back and searched deeper into the mirror for a more familiar self so that I could hold onto reality.

"It's only an outer shell, it's not the real you," I consoled myself and tried to remain calm. "You're okay, you're okay," I repeated. In a split second of panic, I rummaged through the bathroom cabinet for superglue to reassemble the pile of hair that poured over the sides of the wastebasket. But as quickly as the desperate thought came it vanished in a heap of defeat.

Suddenly, Joey appeared in the doorway, "Wow, look at this one," he said as he held up a handful of hair found somewhere between the first and second floor. "This one has three colors." He smiled and spoke as though he just found an autumn leaf. His attempt to minimize the tragedy with light-heartedness helped a bit. I, too, wanted to find humor in the moment, but could only muster up humiliation and embarrassment in large doses.

"Maybe we could make a scrap book," I said, and broke into an incoherent howl. "This is not what I wanted – not even close to what I planned for us." I buried my face in my hands, ashamed of what I'd become, and Joey held me. My feelings went far beyond vanity. As a woman and a new bride, a little sultriness and allure were both parts of the feminine mystique. But now that I had cancer, I felt worthless. At the center of my being, I felt degraded, without entitlement, or purpose enough to walk the earth among able-bodied people. I believed that society marked me as a liability to the healthy. I believed this because at various points in my life I had heard, or known of those sentiments. I didn't want to be sick. I wanted to live, to feel energized, and be beautiful, as society required of me. It was difficult to be any of those things when chemotherapy sheared me to a bloody pulp.

"How can you look at me?" I questioned Joey. "I can't even look at myself right now." I gulped and heaved. "I'm not anything. I'm nothing," I said. "Why do you love me?"

Joey gave a little chuckle. "I'm attracted to you, Michelle - the real you, and not your hair. See?" Joey motioned to his own challenged hairline. "At least your hair is coming back," he said. Still embraced, we looked into the mirror, roared with laughter, and moved past the initial drama of my hair loss.

Later that day, I thought about what Joey said to me in front of the mirror and figured that if he loved me with cancer then I owed it to myself to do the same. It was easier said than done though and would take much more than one conversation for me to erase years of misconceptions and welcome in a more accepting and broader view of myself as a woman and a cancer survivor. Cancer made my insecurities clump together like soured milk and shook the foundation of my beliefs. At thirty-three years old, I thought I had a great deal of self-confidence. Until cancer, I thought I knew my place in the world, what my role was, and what I'd be doing for the next thirty years. The truth was that my scope of myself was too narrow and had no room for my future, not as I saw it, but as it actually would be. I had a lot more to learn about myself, and cancer was my training ground. When my spirits were on empty and my once-grounded philosophies rattled, Joey nudged me forward and sometimes dragged me arm-in-arm up the mountain of my ignorance and disillusionment to find hope. Together we'd peer over the jagged crest to look down upon the greener valleys ahead, but not before I beat myself up over my shortcomings a few hundred times because my definition of a woman never made room for cancer. Like many women, I gave incredible time and effort to an unattainable image of female beauty. If I was a victim of anything, it was society's often false and unjust standards of feminine worth. Matched against cancer, there'd be many re-definitions yet to come.

Though hair loss from chemotherapy is temporary, its loss can pole-vault you to introspection where the truth can be ugly but can also bring permanent self-realizations, if you are willing to look closer. That evening, while I was still stinging from the incident in front of the bathroom mirror, Joey made a bowl of popcorn and we cuddled up on the couch to watch Seinfeld, our favorite television show. My face was bright red and puffy from crying all day. I could tell Joey had a few things on his mind and just wanted to take away my pain.

"I was in my mid- twenties when my hair started to fall out," Joey reminded me. I knew the story and it was an important one for him. "I was very sad," he continued, "my ego couldn't handle it. It was hard to feel good about myself when my outside didn't reflect who I was on the inside and as a man that was very difficult. Professionally, I excelled, but my personal life was terrible. I could hardly get a date. I wanted to be in love, but women only saw me as their friend. I felt like it was all because of my hair loss. Michelle, when I told you this, you said that you didn't care about my hair. I believed you. You saw the real me. You didn't judge me and despite my greatest insecurity I felt free to be myself."

"Yes, absolutely," I said as I trumpeted into a fistful of tissues.

"So why do you think that I would love you less, or not at all, because you are sick and lost your hair from chemo? It hurts my feelings to know that you think that I'm so shallow," he finished.

I was stumped for a logical response and sputtered the first thing that came to mind. "Because, women are supposed to have hair and be beautiful. It's the law." I smiled. Joey gave me a serious look and didn't laugh at my dry humor. I knew that I'd have to get past these issues in order to focus on getting healthy again. I had been forced to anchor myself to this significant yet rocky ideology, but I now had a choice to either slowly tug on this embedded belief, or simply cut the line. While I knew this, I was also a newlywed, and wanted to take advantage of my youthful sexuality.

But the only thing that swung from the chandeliers at that time were my moods from steroids and my hormones from the onset of early menopause due to chemotherapy. No one said anything to me about menopause as a side effect and it went undiagnosed for months. I figured if I had no control over my physical alterations, I'd at least control my reaction to it and maybe in that philosophy I'd gain a new sense of stability. Even though I'd remain challenged for a few months in the hair department, I now felt safer to be myself, at least in my own home. I still had a lot of hills to climb and a great deal of psychological muck to wade through before I'd learn to accept and appreciate my new femininity as a cancer survivor and a valued woman in the world.

Like many people, I associated beauty with health. If you look good and feel good, then it seems unlikely that you'd have a ticking time bomb inside. Right?

My beliefs about womanliness were a product of the generations before me: the mass media and that fast and flashy minority that considers

Hollywood as the compass. Full lips, breasts, and gorgeous hair are always a must have that exudes confidence, sex appeal, and generally amounts to opportunities and success. Throughout time, cultures have reflected these ideas in sculptures, stories, and other artistic expressions. Music, children's fairy tales, and beauty pageants, or as they are more modernly re-packaged, "scholarship pageants," reiterate and reward the beauty ideal. More than ever before, these concepts were difficult to sort through when my mirror reflected a resemblance more in line with Medusa than Sleeping Beauty. Nevertheless, cancer provided me with the opportunity to gain a better comprehension of my intangible qualities. After all, in the end, the measure of a person is judged by words and deeds, not appearances.

Looking back, however, it isn't surprising at all that I was on a perpetual quest for the illusive beauty ideal. Like most women, I always found some grievance about my physical appearance through most stages and ages of my life and saw fat where there was none and a long list of other nonsense. I was never thin, blonde, or sexy enough in my opinion. According to the media no one is, but I wouldn't realize this fact until my thirties. As for my hair maintenance, I'd be rich right now if I had saved that money. Instead, I tried nearly every beauty product with a printed promise in order to achieve perfection. This quest for beauty was apparently a woman's responsibility and as a bride, an even more profound obligation. For months preceding our June Jamaican wedding date I rehearsed the romantic scenes over and over in my head. I was intent on being a picture of loveliness and envisioned misty, cascading stairs and a flowing, chiffon gown with swinging pearls. The dewy, tropical evening air would carry a hint of white gardenias and the melody of soft violins. I imagined that I'd be like some Hollywood screen Goddess from the 1940s, set in radiant lighting, and casting sultry looks at my handsome groom. Dating a year back before our wedding, I began to primp and preen for the big day and gave almost scientific study to bridal magazines that cluttered my house and office. I watched nearly every romantic movie with a wedding theme and my girlfriends and I spent lunch hours at bridal boutiques and weekends at bridal shows. With great excitement I planned every detail.

So, I hired a personal trainer in August of 1999. There'd be no fat on this bride's body. I submitted to a self-prescribed routine that was strict, timed and tactical. The plan began twelve months before the wedding and in reality, decades before the proposal. My trainer was practically an Army boot camp instructor and that's the way I wanted it to be. In our initial meeting, I implored her to not go easy on me. I had a wedding dress to fit into and lifetime portraits to take. As I sculpted my outer appearance, I didn't know that my greatest imperfection lay between my lungs, unnoticed by the world around me.

"Give me ten more," she demanded, "C'mon, I'll count you down." Sweat stung my eyes as I took in a deep breath and gave her all the physical power I possessed. Just as I neared the end of the set, she'd bellow out, "Okay, now give me three more. Can you feel the burn? Don't stop now. C'mon, Michelle you can do it!" She'd shout out, "Push it…push it…push it!" like I was having a baby or something. In my head I'd scream a silent litany of profanities, vowed that I hated her, and reminded myself why I paid for such abuse in the first place. I'd always go the distance with my trainer and after every workout, I felt strong and alive in the rush of endorphin highs that followed. As tough as those workouts were, they paled in comparison to the sum total of mind, body, and spiritual endurance I'd need to battle and cope with cancer.

Also included in my quest for wedding day perfection were twelve micro-dermabrasion sessions, or as I like to call them, facial sandblasting – it was hardly a blast. This painful process strips away the top layer of skin that can reveal a woman's age. With an instrument as small as a pencil but as brutal as a floor sander, my face was traced like a jack-o-lantern on a weekly basis for months. No furrowed lines could escape the cruelty. I winced with pain, swallowed my curse words, and bit my lip to avoid screaming throughout the salon.

Despite the discomfort, I remained undeterred in my pursuits and continued with other regular beauty treatments that included: teeth whitening, weekly manicures, pedicures, eyebrow tweezing, and torturous leg waxing. For weeks my hair stylist and I scoured through armfuls of magazines as we laughed, gossiped, and slurped gallons of iced caramel and mocha frappes. We debated over wearing it up, down, with curls, or loosely pinned around my rhinestone tiara and opted for the later. My walk down the aisle would, after all, be the moment of all moments; cameras would snap to capture a temporary moment for a lifetime of reflection. Just a few weeks into chemotherapy, much of the beauty quest seemed a sad and wasted effort when I realized that Joey loved me as I was and that my greatest imperfection threatened my life each day.

***

<u>May 11, 2000</u>

I'm exhausted. Short of breath. 3000 white blood count. Stomach pains. Are we having fun yet?

<u>May 14, 2000</u>

Joey and I went to the mall today. I dragged my body around like a zombie with barely enough energy to walk the first floor. The anemia from chemo makes my body feel three times heavier. It's hard to stay motivated when I have no energy. Tomorrow I go back to work after being out a couple of weeks. I need normalcy back in my life and going to work every day will do the trick for me. Of course I don't look forward to all of the cancer related talk that will ensue: the talk of religion, nutrition and other such stories. I don't want other people's opinions right now. I need to stay in my own head.

***

Within the first few weeks of chemo, my sensibilities were awakened with several profound realizations, which proved to be the best coping strategies for me over the years of my illness. I've always had good sense of humor, adored all kinds of comedy, and realized that humor was as important to me as the chemotherapy that I took to survive. One day, I orchestrated some needed comic relief to endure the conflicted idea of intentional poisoning by chemotherapy. I strolled into the oncology office with a magic wand. A rhinestone tiara twinkled on top of my head and a neon pink feather boa draped to the floor. I announced to the staff that I was the "Queen of Chemotherapy" and they were the "Cancer Divas." Since they were a zany bunch without my help, they instantly took to my brand of humor. Not only were chemo cocktails served up that day, but lots of laughter too. Throughout the afternoon, the magic wand waved to cast a variety of fairy Godmother spells and many other hilarious make-believe wishes. We each took turns wearing the boa and tiara, and walked an imaginary fashion runway in the chemo room as we said, "How do I look, Dah-ling?" Pink feathers flew into the air and from nowhere, Dr. Smith appeared. His gaze narrowed at the scene before him as he watched his staff and I behave like six-year-olds at a tea party. He said nothing and shook his head as if helpless to our silly antics, which made us all burst out with even more laughter. But despite the laughter that day, I still stirred with many concerns and questions.

No matter how much humor filled a day, there were many difficult days ahead with no humor to be found when Death tapped me on the shoulder as a reminder. I wasn't ready to die. On some days my faith was shaken, and I was so pissed off that heaven probably wouldn't have let me in. The phrase "War on Cancer" resonated with me and baffled me too. It was vague, faceless, and a cultural cliché, similar to "a thousand points of light" or "speak softly and carry a big stick." It was all embedded rhetoric and I fully understood none of it. I fought for my life and didn't want to hear media quips. I knew that science had come a long way but people still died from cancer. In an effort to cope, I longed to find an understandable context within the intangible swirl. What special significance did the "War on Cancer" phrase contain when war battles played out in precise images on the evening news and were further described as being "like a cancer?" What was the image of the War on Cancer anyway; obscure research labs and thirty-second news stories about possible cures twenty years away? I had cancer right now. And what about the profiteers who got rich off the misfortunes of others? Was that the War on Cancer, too?

With these questions, a series of other questions emerged for me. Where did the diagnosed, the cured and the deceased fit into the war concept? Was our role as patients to be voiceless bystanders, un-empowered victims, and undirected until some remote research lab discovered "a cure"? Is that when we'd live again and find happiness for ourselves? I wanted to live happy right now in spite of cancer. What was the unifying, symbolic image of the War on Cancer and if there was one, was it effective? Which weapons hadn't we considered? Throughout my cancer battle I'd continue to participate in and advocate for cancer research. However, I also recognized that the power of science alone could not ever fill me with enough daily hope, courage, inspiration, or humor to cope with cancer. In the darkest moments of fear and despair, no cancer researcher came to my bedside to encourage me to fight harder and celebrate my small victories. No lab helped me with insurance forms, informed me about my employee rights, counseled, or educated me about early menopause, infertility, my changed body image, and purpose in the world. Nor, would research directly console the thousands of grieving families and offer them a tangible place of remembrance, honor, and retreat.

History teaches that wars are never won with a single weapon. Education, prevention, awareness, and psychosocial tools are also powerful weapons and together, work to surround and defeat the enemy's power. A pistol fired into the air sends caution to an opponent, but relentless firepower is a planned tactic used to destroy the enemy and win the war. From the first moments of my diagnosis, the phrase "War on Cancer" echoed in my ears like a primal drumbeat, and continued to signal me onward in my search for answers and to the source of my greatest epiphany.

I was now two months into my cancer journey and for the most part had settled into the routine and was finding my way through the mire. I still had moments of denial about the fact that I had cancer, but realized that in addition to the term cancer victim, the term cancer patient also unsettled me. I'm a cancer survivor and for me, this point is the critical difference between being passive or proactive about my health. As long as my heart beats, I am alive and that truth makes me a survivor. I can't control whether or not I have cancer, but I can control my perception of myself within it. Chemo on the other hand, was a more cumbersome issue to mentally overcome and it physically robbed me of normal amounts of red blood cells. As a result, it soon became impossible to keep up with a normal pace. I was stunned to realize the power of chemotherapy drugs. Nothing in nature compares to the physical beat down that it delivers to every bodily cell. I was incredibly fatigued, dizzy, and short-winded. For a while, I worked every day, but it soon became a struggle to last until five o'clock and then commute forty-minutes back home in rush-hour traffic. My workouts at the gym were soon down to once a week. As a result, the lack of endorphin highs was a difficult adjustment for my body and mind. Moments of depression and doubt swept in and out so I wrote in my journal a lot just to keep my thoughts together.

During the first couple of weeks of daily visits to the cancer center, I observed other cancer survivors and accepted that I was now a part of the group. Some were visibly weakened by their illness and others weren't. Some people still had hair; others didn't and didn't seem to care about it either. Each week I'd see familiar faces and became friends with many. The diagnosed were people of all backgrounds, ages, and professions: teachers, mechanics, business executives, mothers with young children, and dads who were their family's only source of income. One thing I couldn't blame cancer for was discrimination. Some people traveled across several states for their chemotherapy. Three or four generations congregated just to hold the hand of a loved one and together they'd cope through the ordeal. I was unprepared to see so much love in one room. It was beautiful.

Other than my friend Maureen, I'd never been around someone with cancer and hadn't ever stepped foot in a cancer center. Collectively,

I'd only heard negative stereotypes of what cancer patients were supposed to look or be like, but now in front of me were crowds of people with cancer, just like me. Where once I peddled along in my ideas about cancer, now I could scarcely contain the light speed at which old and new thoughts merged. These were ordinary, everyday people who paid their taxes, voted, and did their own grocery shopping. They had worked for decades and now this. These folks didn't live to be rich. They raised their children to be good citizens and struggled to provide a safe, loving home. They enjoyed laughter with friends and family at weekend barbeques, and hoped to have enough money to retire comfortably. There was no self-pity at the cancer center. I saw no victims. Instead, I saw courage in spite of fear and tremendous hope in the face of the unknown. I was inspired to know them all. Despite their cancer diagnosis and tears of confusion, each person that I talked to continued to live with great joy and purpose. They were in the pursuit of life, not waiting to die. They planned for upcoming birthday parties, holiday celebrations, and vacations.

In the most unlikely place, I found my muse and the dormant creativity was re-awakened within me. I learned their stories and we spoke on the deepest of levels that such a crisis permits. Our conversations got right to the core of what it means to be human. There was no pretense or competition. With cancer, now there was time only for truth. The experience was more than any college philosophy class ever offered me and filled me with immense inspiration. From each person, I learned something that helped me cope with my own battle and the humor of those conversations left me laughing for hours and sometimes days later. These weren't victims by a long shot. I swelled with immense pride for this uncelebrated humanity of which I now belonged. Beyond the walls of the cancer center, I knew that millions more battled cancer with courage, valor, and some to their death. Each had a story of hope and inspiration, but for us all there remained an immense need to cope with the daily uncertainties of life without a cure.

A big question suddenly jabbed at my heart. Who will tell their stories? I searched for a way to capture and display this powerful information and knew that if I was inspired, others would be as well, and that alone might make the difference between life and death for someone. Verbal or written forms had been my usual mediums of creative expression, but this was beyond words. My thoughts and feelings built inside me with no proper outlet, but an answer was on its way.

***

I didn't have God on my speed dial, but we were on good terms. I'd been too busy in the weeks following my cancer diagnosis and wedding ceremony to remember that prayer was a coping option and I was now overdue for a conversation with the big guy upstairs.

Alone, I stood in my living room one day and began to pray out loud, "God, you've got to help me out here because I don't know how to get through this. I don't blame you for my cancer, but I need to find the purpose and meaning behind it all. Use me. Use me, God. Help me to understand and if in some way I can help other people then that will be great, too."

And there it was. I gave an open invitation for what was about to happen to me next. I opened my eyes and at that precise moment a television news clip about the Vietnam Memorial played. Like a lightning bolt, the vision of what would become The Cancer Monument struck. My vision lasted no more than a second, but within that time, an eternity of information was given to me. It revealed a monument to honor and celebrate the hope, courage, and inspiration of ageless, timeless, unsung heroes in the War on Cancer. The living and the dead, ranked side by side without prejudice in a mighty show of legendary force that would loudly proclaim many messages to the world. I saw the monument in a circular shape like that of a human cell. The walls were very big and emanated a vibrant force, which held thousands of inscribed names. Waves of people stood before it with great emotion. I knew that this was my answer. Uncontained excitement ran through my body unlike anything I had felt before.

Tears streamed as I jumped up and down in my living room and shouted, "I'm building a monument, I'm building a monument! If this is a War on Cancer, then those who battle it are soldiers. Where is our monument to honor our heroes?" Breathing hard, I reached for the phone to call Joey at work. I bubbled over with excitement before he had a chance to say hello.

"But Michelle, you have cancer," he reminded. "How are you going to build a monument?"

"I'll figure it out, and so what I have cancer," I shrugged. "When is a good time to build a monument anyway?" I asked. "All wars end at some point and this one hasn't. It has to be built, and it's not about you, or me. This is about a War on Cancer and its unsung heroes. If I don't build it, who will? The image of the victim must be transformed into hero status. This monument will be that story."

Joey and I talked about how the monument would be a landmark;

a beacon, a place to raise more money for research, not just for a day, or a weekend, but for the generations. We talked about how the monument would educate, inspire and bring hope to those who need it most. I told Joey about what I'd seen in my vision, about the 60,000 names that would be inscribed on granite walls and how each inscribed name would serve as a symbolic ambassador for millions more who have battled cancer, do battle, and those who will battle.

"Who qualifies as a hero?" Joey asked.

"Anyone who has battled cancer?" I said.

"Even those who died?"

"Absolutely," I said. "If a soldier dies in battle, are they stripped of medals and dishonored?" I asked.

Joey laughed through his words. "No, not at all," he said. "Never. But, what's hopeful about a person who died from cancer?"

Joey and I talked about the meaning of the word hope and how it has a different meaning for each person. We talked about how important it is to see those with cancer as heroes instead of victims and how the power of those ideas and a monument can teach and inspire generations. I was bursting with new passion. "I want to shake people up and say, 'Hey, look over here, now put that cigarette down once and for all'. I want people to approach this massive monument and say, 'Aha! I get it now'." Everything just poured out of me as if I had always known it. "It's time for something unconventional," I insisted.

"Well, you've never been ordinary, that's for sure, but that's part of your charm," Joey chimed.

"Joey," I said, "this monument will be prolific and there will be nothing like it anywhere."

"If you build it they will come," Joey said, like Kevin Costner in the movie, Field of Dreams. "Will it make you happy to see it built?"

"It makes me happy already," I said.

"Okay, then you know I'll be behind you one hundred percent."

I now had the answer that I longed for – The Cancer Monument. With it, I had a purpose to get out of bed on the worst days of my life. I didn't know what the future held for me. Maybe this was all the life I'd get. I planned to live it to the fullest and not be held hostage by fear. I was a soldier in the War on Cancer and if winning meant a flesh-tearing, tooth-spitting, bloody showdown in the trenches, I was ready for it. I'd fight cancer anywhere, anyhow, whether a bar room brawl, or a back alley down and dirty, my cancer cells would no longer be confused about who was in charge.

"Is that all the muscle you've got, wimp? I'm about to drop a bomb on you like a nuclear winter," I'd say to my cancer cells. Since I was in charge of these mental fantasies, I never gave cancer the power to talk back. I couldn't imagine that it'd have anything smart to say, anyway. On many days, I'd throw mental punches at my cancer and imagined the success of a relentless southpaw hook, below the belt, and upper cut combination. And just to thumb my nose at cancer and its attempts to limit me and wreak a mighty hell on the rest of us, I vowed to build The Cancer Monument despite my cancer diagnosis. If I could help it, I wouldn't delay one single moment of time. The Cancer Monument and I now journeyed together towards wholeness, purpose, and life.

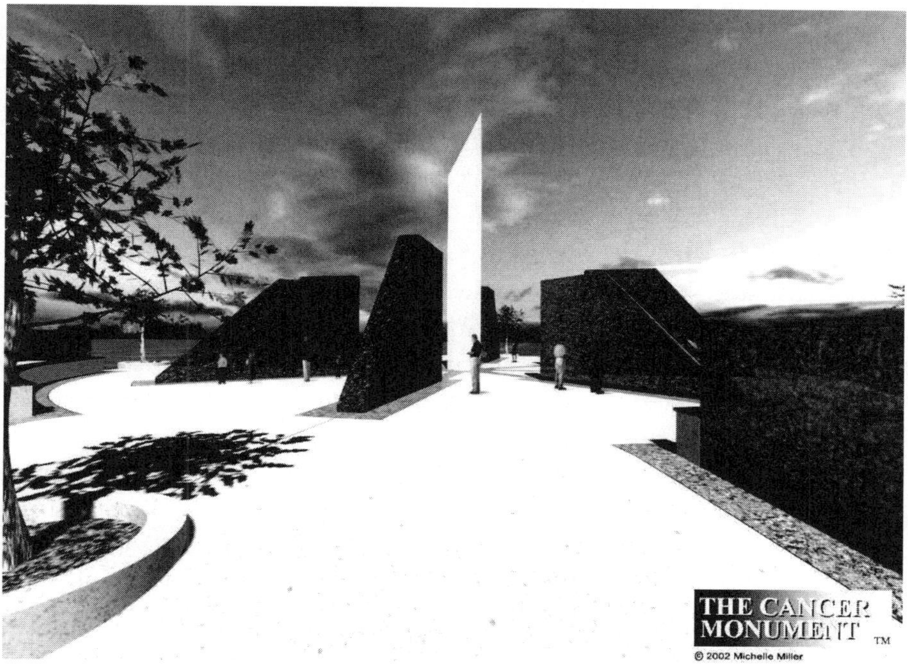

"You gain strength, courage and confidence by every experience in which you really stop to look fear in the face. You are able to say to yourself, 'I have lived through this horror. I can take the next thing that comes along.' You must do the thing you think you cannot do."

—Eleanor Roosevelt

Chapter 2
Soldiers Are Made

Looking back, it's as though I've trained my entire life for this brief window of time, so The Cancer Monument can be built. Fate plopped me down in the middle of this cancer battleground. The soldier analogy occurred to me early in my fight. It first pounded in my head like rapid cannon fire and was then followed by the vision of The Cancer Monument. In the first year of battle, I shared my monument idea in depth with only the closest people in my life. They all said the same thing to me. 'Put cancer behind you and then work on the monument.' I didn't listen. The Cancer Monument couldn't wait. It had been needed for so long and now, although only in my mind, it was real. Its presence was among us and demanded to be built.

In the solitary moments of the first fourteen months of my cancer, the monument mostly stayed in my head and went no further than the rough proposals and sketches that I drafted. With each step, I stayed true to the monument's design concept, symbolism, and the driving purpose behind it, as it was revealed to me on that momentous day in my living room. At that time, I knew nothing about politics, bureaucracy, or non-profit business. The fact that I'd have to start and become the president of a non-profit organization in order to build the monument was at first an intimidating prospect, but soon became a natural way of being. No matter how sick I was in the years ahead, the vision of the monument and the very papers that contained its future comforted me like an angel. However, as my physical state became weakened by chemotherapy, the art and strategy of daily coping required creative measures beyond the promise of the monument.

On many days, I fought my cancer cells with large doses of creative visualization. I imagined a variety of battle scenes between cancer and me. I was a soldier and wore full combat gear with rows of bullets across my chest, and knives strategically located as back-up weaponry. I was a one-woman arsenal and ready to annihilate the enemy. There'd be no retreat from my end of the fight. Muddied but strong, I'd crawl under razor sharp wires through open stretches of dark, dry earth. Acrid smoke filled the air and burned my eyes. I always knew where to find the black-celled enemy, as I'd canvass the landscape of my internal organs and lymphatic system. Afraid to stand alone, they'd always travel in groups; the dark cowards realized that their safety was in numbers. My mouth tasted of bitter gunpowder and was too dry to spit, but my stealth was undeterred. Now safely through a thicket of wires, there were no hills, forests, or grasslands to protect me as I ran across the battlefield. An explosion of grenades and missiles could be felt at the pit of my stomach and at times was so close that I was lifted off the ground. Mud caked my ears but did not minimize the sound of bullets that flew by within inches of my head. With the enemy in view, I'd run to a full-on attack and spared no mercy as thousands of determined cancer cells shook with fear at the sight of my crazed approach. When my ammunition ran out, I'd resort to hand-to-hand combat and took back territory within me from this ancient infiltrator whose sole mission is to destroy me, and everything in its path. With my sword held high in the air, I'd stand atop ashen cells and was ready to wage more war against cancer. In the long dark, lonely times when all I could do was lay, think, hope, and pray that Western medicine would work for me, I'd envision myself the victor of these imagined scenes.

The soldier tactic was familiar, comfortable, and appropriate for me. Many might wonder how this intense coping strategy emerged so quickly, but it's easy to understand when you know more about my life before cancer. My first lessons in battle tactics came long before I ever received a cancer diagnosis. I can scarcely remember a time when the adults in my family didn't speak about heavy issues like war at back yard barbeques, holidays, or weddings. Wherever two or more of us gathered, chances were great that three sides of a State Of The Union address were up for debate. Someone in our family was always in the military so discussions either began or ended with military talk, which yielded other current and intense topics such as politics, crime, or the welfare system. All were served up in loud, heavy portions to young and old alike along with the potato salad, burgers, hot dogs, and apple pie.

A family history on my maternal grandmother's side dates back to the 1600s and also includes stories of patriotism from the Revolutionary War. In more recent decades, my uncle, three brothers, cousins, and a few close friends of the family all served in various branches of the military and many saw real combat in World War II, Vietnam, the jungles of Central America, Afghanistan, and Iraq. Over the years, these first-hand war accounts taught me many physical and psychological lessons of survival that as a child, I first acted out in play with my brother Mike and eventually applied to the real world and the War on Cancer.

We lived on a street called Miller Circle in the rural town of Newburgh, New York, situated between the Hudson and Wallkill Rivers and just seventy miles north of New York City. Growing up, family day trips included all sorts of museums as well as West Point Military Academy and many nearby historic battle sites of the Revolutionary War period. They lined the banks of the Hudson River and included General Washington's Headquarters, Knox Headquarters and the New Windsor Cantonment, which was the site of the final winter encampment of the Washington-led Continental Army. Stewart Air Force Base, now called Stewart International Airport, is also located in Newburgh and was the site of a few air shows that I went to when I was a kid. I'll never forget the experience of being inside the body of a military cargo plane that could hold several buses and still have lots of room left over. So, before the age of ten I'd seen many war reenactments, felt the raw, thunderous power of military machines and understood patriotism as much as is possible for a child. Our grandparents on both sides infused us with the heroic stories of our relatives in combat.

"Your grandfather was a hero in World War II and received the Purple Heart," my grandmother Miller told my brother Mike and me.

"What's a Purple Heart?" we asked. Grandma Miller liked to tell us the battle stories from WW II and we loved to hear them, because she always gave lots of details that made us feel like we were really there. As she'd knit, Mike and I sat on her dark blue living room carpet, and looked up at her with open-mouthed anticipation for the next detail that could spark ten new questions from each of us.

"What did the German soldiers look like? Did Grandpa have a bayonet? Did he throw hand grenades? How many enemies did he kill? Did he sleep in a tent? What did the soldiers eat?" we'd shout out before she could finish the next sentence. Like it all happened yesterday, Grandma Miller answered every question and told us about courageous battles scenes on the beaches of Normandy and on the farms and towns of France and Germany.

Born and raised in the Bronx, Grandma Miller was a young lady in love who awaited her hero's return. Grandpa came back from the war, as did many other uncles and cousins, but many men didn't and she always remembered them and said a prayer. She also told us about the glories of victory, how thousands of people kissed and danced in the streets of New York City, and of the great ticker tape parades down 5th Avenue. Then she'd show us grandpa's Purple Heart. It was a thrill to touch it and to know that it once hung on his chest. Grandpa Miller never got to show us his battle wounds because he died in a car accident a little more than a decade after the war. My grandmother raised their four children on her own and never remarried.

Through the words and passion of my grandmother, Mike and I learned history and grew to know and love the courageous, and honorable man who was our grandfather. My other grandfather, Ernest Brown on the maternal side, belonged to the homeland security brigade during World War II and was a lookout for enemy planes. After the war, the Cold War posed serious threats for an atomic collision with Russia, then known as the Soviet Union. So, my grandfather designed and constructed a bomb shelter in the basement of their home on Harrison Street that was big enough for their family of seven. For many decades in the village of Walden, New York, my grandparents were newsworthy for their numerous charitable works, but in the late 1950s their bomb shelter was the talk of the town and the local Citizen Herald newspaper. Of course, as history proved, the bomb shelter was never needed and who knows if it, or its inhabitants, could've endured an actual air raid or atomic blast. After the threat of war subsided the bomb shelter was turned into a spare bedroom and decades later, it gave Mike and me the perfect atmosphere to play out all kinds of imagined war battles.

Even though Mike was a year younger than me, I was by no means "the boss" of him. For certain, he wasn't going to play with dolls, so I ended up playing with trucks and toy soldiers. As little kids, it was an ironclad law that we were not allowed to play inside the bomb shelter at all. Rightly so, the adults always imagined the worst and were afraid that we'd get locked behind the heavy steel door, suffocate, and die. Mike and I had an adventurous streak and the taboo only served to increase our insatiable desire to tempt fate, if only to stick a toe inside the bomb shelter and re-enact battle scenes that we'd seen on the evening news about the war in Vietnam. With the song of the show Mission Impossible on our lips, Mike and I planned our mission to sneak down to my grandparents' basement as soon as we were sure that the adults were distracted. Sometimes our plan was foiled at the turn of the basement doorknob as the grownups possessed super hearing abilities far beyond what our plan allowed.

"Don't you two go near that bomb shelter. Stay out of the basement. How many times do I have to tell you?" they'd warn us with stern voices and layered threats. Other times we made it past the doorknob phase, but were betrayed by the creaking sound of the basement door. On enough occasions however, we accomplished our mission because everyone was too busy to hear, or notice our absence, at least for a while anyway. Once in the basement our minds transported to the wondrous magic of imagination as we touched the big, heavy steel door, and stepped inside the bomb shelter.

"Our plane is hit," Mike said, "we have to eject and parachute down to find our troops." Of course, our troops were located, where else but the safety of the bomb shelter. We'd pretend to be thrown in the air by the force of the ejection and then wafted down to earth in our parachutes. The entire way down, we imagined airplane battles above our heads and Mike made the sounds of rapid gunfire, diving aircraft, and explosions. Sometimes, to increase the drama, a bullet would injure one of us. Still parachuting down, Mike would call out to me, "I've been shot in the leg, we've got to radio for an ambulance to meet us on the ground."

"No," I'd call back. The sound of explosions overhead forced us to yell out to one another in the sky. "There are no ambulances, when we get to the ground, we've got to run for it and try to find the bomb shelter. That's were our men are."

"Okay, but enemy tanks are everywhere," he'd say.

Even as a kid, Mike loved danger and always pushed the limits of imagination and possibility. It wasn't enough for him to be ejected from a plane, shot in the leg and have to run to find the safety of some obscure bomb shelter through the maze of a battlefield; he had to be surrounded by enemy tanks too and take me with him. But, war games taught me a lot. I learned the art of the quiet stalk. Even pretend war had a lot of rules and could get downright nasty. We tried to make our wars a fair battle and discussed what types of weapons were allowed so that no one had more firepower than the next guy. Sometimes, if you were captured you might be shot and out of the game, or you might be taken prisoner and forced to fight on the opposite team. After being shot or captured too many times, I learned how to avoid "the enemy". I climbed trees, or hid in ambush under leaves and bushes like my opponents did.

On an instinctual level some of these early lessons about how to survive seemed like basic common sense mixed with fun. Later on, I realized that though survival was a primary goal of war, it was dependent on many factors, not all of which are predictable or fair. As a soldier, it's not enough to maneuver and outwit seen and unseen enemies; you have to think like the enemy if you live in the combat zone. From my cousins and brothers in the military, I learned the stories of some who never made it out of basic training and others who didn't survive the first days of battle. The gentle ones, those in denial, the conscientious observers, the unarmed, the naive, or the shell-shocked never stood a chance against the realities of war.

Those were difficult concepts for me to absorb at a young age since I was taught that good always outweighed bad. But, in order to win against a non-negotiable force such as cancer that didn't value human life, or abide by any ethical standards, I'd have to quickly adjust to the crisis or be devoured by it. First, I'd have to accept the challenge of battle and wear the truth of my reality like a uniform. Then, I'd have to study the enemy, arm myself, out maneuver, and maintain my march towards victory.

***

For many years, I only knew my Uncle Gene through family stories and the many pictures that adorned my grandparents' house. "Your Uncle Gene is a hero," Grandma Brown would say to Mike and me as we made paper airplanes and acted out air raids in her kitchen as she cooked. My grandmother beamed with a mixture of pride and a look of distant sadness as she spoke of her oldest son who was half a world away in Vietnam. My uncle was a Navy fighter pilot and flew many missions over enemy territory. In one photograph, Uncle Gene stood in his Navy uniform next to a fighter jet and in another he was in the cockpit and saluted to the camera with a great smile.

These stories and pictures filled Mike and me with pride as well as many questions: Where was Vietnam? Why was there a war and when could we see Uncle Gene? My grandmother explained war as best as one can to young children and said that my uncle protected our freedom and would be home soon.

Somehow I made the connection that the war my uncle fought on the other side of the world, tied in with the practice air raid drills that we had at my elementary school. As we sat at our desks in the middle of a lesson, the alarm bell rang, and the loud speaker told us that it was only a drill. The teacher's face always looked strained on these occasions but we soon learned that calm and orderliness were required in emergency situations. The entire school, including the janitor, crammed into the basement as we stood in forced silence while the adults checked their watches. These routine drills stopped around fourth grade. My uncle came back from the war and it was a thrill to finally meet the handsome, tall, white-uniformed man that I'd only seen in photographs. After the war, my uncle was a candidate for the NASA astronaut program, but an accelerated heartbeat eventually prevented him from continuing further. Until retirement, he continued his flying career as a private pilot and to this day Mike and I idolize our Uncle Gene.

As you enter the town of Walden, a large bronze statue of President William McKinley presides at the fork in the road. According to our family history, William McKinley, the twenty-fifth U.S. president, was a cousin to us through marriage on my maternal grandmother's side. From the backseat of the station wagon Mike and I bounced with excited pride to wave at President McKinley and say, "Hi, cuz!"

For generations most of my relatives came from a long line of Pennsylvania and New York farmers, mostly dairy, and a few were independent merchants. Over the years I've tended to a good amount of chickens, goats, and cows, churned butter till I thought my arms would fall off, baked bread, and picked heaping baskets of strawberries until I thought I'd never wanted to eat another. I've baled hay, shoveled piles of crap out of the barn, hauled and stacked firewood, mixed cement and laid brick, too.

Along with the day-to-day of rural life, other survival lessons were taught in the process. Responsibility, respect for the land and a great deal of independence came with a good dose of humility. Everyone eats a little dirt from time to time while weeding, hoeing, and vying against swarms of hungry mosquitoes in the garden. Everyone was expected to do a fair share of work and no red carpets were rolled out for anyone when a harvest of vegetables had to be canned, frozen, or pickled. In the winter, each had their turn at shoveling hip-deep snow from our very long driveway. Resourcefulness, perseverance, and cooperation were the result of routine chores and are also the qualities needed in situations of crisis. When we ran out of ideas for zucchinis and tomatoes they made their way into breads and preserves.

Knowledge, respect and a little fear for weaponry were in good measure. Since my father belonged to a hunting club, I learned not only how to fish, but how to gut and clean them, too, as well as to be comfortable around guns. Around ten years old, I felt the powerful force behind a trigger and shot many types of rifles and handguns under the watchful eye of my father and the cautionary words of my mother, "Don't shoot your eye out."

By age twelve, I was as good a shot with a gun as some of the men in my father's hunting club, who were a bunch of sore heads one day when I almost won the skeet shooting contest.

***

President Nixon declared "War on Cancer" in the 1970's. Like the rest of America, I'd hear that "War on Cancer" phrase a thousand times over the decades and never did it become any more visual or defined. I didn't know the meaning of rhetoric then, so after hearing the news state that war was like a cancer, I figured that cancer must be the worst of all. Eventually, I'd learn the truth for myself, but until then, I was a voracious reader who loved history and was content to be alone with a set of encyclopedias for hours or at the old upright piano in the basement.

When the adults talked, I took greater enjoyment at listening to and participating in their conversations about large ideas and concepts than any kid games. I'd always throw my two cents worth into their conversation and much to their surprise they didn't know that a child could have such big opinions. But I did and turned out to be a studious kid who was well liked by many teachers, classmates and was voted school vice president in my eleventh grade year. I excelled in the social sciences, literature, music, and foreign language. From sixth grade on I was involved in the school music program, student government, and cheerleading.

I could be a little unruly at times like in the fourth grade when I gave a fifth grade boy twice my size a black eye for picking on my brother. Once in middle school, I almost got kicked off the school bus for a compilation of minor infractions and along the way, I did a fair share of mouthing-off to a few teachers and was sent to the principal's office or detention. Around eighth grade, the ego of an all-too-important school social life took center stage and gave me no time or interest for the un-cool consequences of bad behavior.

I had lots of friends throughout school; Maureen, Yvonne, Maria and Ginny were my best friends. At Yvonne's house I learned to ride horses and drive a car. We'd take her parents' old station wagon into the open riding fields behind the barn and practice in anticipation of a learner's permit still a couple of years away. At Maureen's house, I perfected my cannonballs and belly flops in their pool. Maureen was an excellent swimmer and beat me every time in a race. She was proud to be of Irish blood and said that her grandparents were "from the four corners of Ireland." St. Patrick's Day was a huge day of celebration for the McVeigh family. Her father was a New York City fire fighter, stationed in the Bronx. He'd come home on the weekends, exhausted, his face red from the intensity of heat, and black soot still on his hands. From time to time, he'd tell us the courageous stories of the men in his firehouse, some we even saw on the evening news.

In eighth grade, my prayers to God were for the continuous life of the disco phase. I still had several years to go before I was of legal age to boogie my fever nights away at Studio 54 in Manhattan, only 70 miles south.

In homeroom one morning, Maureen let me know that in her opinion, disco sucked and rock and roll was forever. "Who cares about the Village People and Sister Sledge when there's Lynyrd Skynyrd, the Rolling Stones and the Grateful Dead," she said.

"Disco lives," I proclaimed.

"Rock and roll is forever," Maureen held up her fist in protest.

We went back and forth and finally decided to put democracy to work and conducted a poll of the class. The results were split.

It would be years more before I'd live in New York City, and even though I looked forward to the excitement, I knew that it was a different life than the rural one I knew. Every night on the evening news I saw glimpses of that cosmopolitan and dangerous world and even saw it first hand on school trips to Broadway shows, museums, and Fifth Avenue parades. As we played patriotic tunes, drunks grabbed our rear ends; our bandleader, Mr. Izzo beat them off with his megaphone.

Eventually, the disco heat fizzled and punk rock led one of the new music scenes of the 1980s. Being a country girl, the daily sight of a true punk rocker was non-existent, but we had the watered-down version of wanna-be punkers at Wallkill High School, at least as much as the rules would permit. School policy made it difficult for any student to look like a true punk rocker. Chains, studded leather bracelets, crazy hair, and ripped clothing wasn't allowed and resulted in suspension if worn.

The Manhattan Punk scene was the real deal with their serious attitudes, leather outfits, wildly spiked hair, and chains that attached from nose to ear. Their appearance reflected the social and political issues of the day: drugs, unemployment, homelessness, and the threat of nuclear war with the Soviet Union. Maybe the punkers figured since the world would end in 1984, as the doomsayers predicted, nothing mattered anyway.

For me, an impressionable teenager, it was a curious sight to see anti-establishment twenty-somethings strut along the Manhattan streets with steel-toed boots and a cocky air as if to challenge the world to knock the big chip off their shoulder. My friends and I wouldn't dream of teasing them from street level, but we heckled them plenty from the safe confines of the school bus window as we inched through downtown traffic. In all aspects, city life and its inhabitants were an intrigue, and as I got older, it was apparent that I wouldn't find my opportunities around Newburgh. Making the switch to city life would be a brave step forward and took careful planning.

After graduation, I worked a year or so at radio station WGNY in Newburgh, where I wrote commercials during the week for minimum wage and snapped up the opportunity to be a radio host for the early morning weekend drives that no one else wanted. I was eighteen years old, had my own radio show, and went to college full time at Orange County Community College.

Many of my friends left for college in other states. Maureen went to school in Florida to study marine biology and she'd phone me with stories of her dive adventures inside sunken ships and awesome parties full of gorgeous, fun, polite guys in Key West and in Fort Lauderdale. She'd periodically return to New York to visit and one night we saw Prince in concert at Madison Square Garden and sang along to every song.

Unlike my friends, I found little time for parties. I studied and had to be at the radio station by 4:30 a.m. to work for $3.35 an hour. Minimum wage hardly bought the basics, but the experience at the radio station was great. One day, one of my co-workers talked very excitedly about his new part-time real-estate career. Before I knew it, I too found my way into real estate and first learned the ropes in the area of mortgage finance with a company in Westchester. Now that I made more than minimum wage, I inched my way closer to the city and eventually moved to the borough of Queens. Safe areas with quality apartments were few in New York City during the late 1980s, which made finding an affordable place to live even more difficult. I was ecstatic to find a terrific duplex apartment off Steinway Street in Astoria for $900 a month that would've cost three times more if it had been fifteen minutes away in Manhattan. I had the most fabulous view of the Manhattan skyline and was only a short cab ride to LaGuardia Community College where I attended classes.

For the first year, I loved city life and experienced all that it had to offer, but slowly, the urban jungle took its toll, and daily life in New York City became a struggle. The problems of city life were endless. Blazing hot summers had humidity enough to choke the life out of you. Roads, sidewalks, and black-tar rooftops baked during the day, and barely cooled by nightfall. Electricity rates were so high that you couldn't afford to keep yourself cool. Garbage bags and cans lined the streets and were knocked over, ripped open by hungry dogs, or bums. If not picked up regularly in the summer, the fermented rot produced a horrid stench that forced you to stay inside or run down the street holding your breath until you'd gasp for air. In the winter, the snowy streets could remain unplowed for days and if you didn't remember exactly where the enormous potholes were, you'd risk serious damage to your car.

Finding a place to park on the street was another problem. As a car owner, I risked theft or damage daily. Just because you found a great spot on one day, didn't mean that you'd keep it the next. All street parking spaces were fair game and could easily erupt in shouting matches and fistfights when in dispute. The worst were the double parkers, who blocked you in because they were too rude and lazy to find a legitimate parking space on the next block over. The street sweeper laws were another hassle. No matter the weather, and even if monster snowplow trucks buried your car, you had to dig out, move your vehicle or get a ticket.

The noise of city life was constant; trains went by every fifteen minutes and taxicabs honked at all hours. Brazen rats, usually known to be nocturnal creatures, grew as big as alley cats, and showed no fear of humans and on occasion were known to attack in broad daylight. Unsafe people of all varieties roamed the streets at all hours: drug addicts, the insane, violent criminals, or just common street hustlers. The general atmosphere and level of cautiousness produced sometimes hostile and almost always, superficial relationships between people. I felt sorry for kids who had nowhere to play except in the streets or on playgrounds with broken swings, broken glass, and where drug dealers roamed to turn a wide-eyed youngster into a new customer. In the summer, open fire hydrants provided the only means of water recreation for city kids.

As I'd watch from my terrace, I thought about the children that I might have one day and knew even more that life in the city would be temporary. I didn't like walking down the street with my keys positioned between my fingers ready to counter-attack at a moment's notice, but it was an unavoidable part of city life and I'd have been an easy target to believe otherwise. Out on the open jungle streets, in my car, even in my apartment, I no longer had the benefit of innocence, which might easily be spotted by a human beast ready to pounce on its prey. As a long-term way of life, the big city was out of balance and not for me. For my survival, I acquired a cynical view of people. It never existed before, but slowly, caution embedded into my bones and emerged through my personality. I had an acute case of street smarts. It didn't feel good at all.

For the most part, I enjoyed my work in the mortgage business especially when I had my commission check in hand. But then, the stock market crash of 1987 left real estate markets on shaky ground. While many lost their jobs and homes, others with a little bit of capital played a real life game of Monopoly. Within the next three years, I acquired three rental properties and with it became the landlord for twenty-one apartments, which added at least forty new complaints a week on my to-do list. For a while, I handled all the property management issues, but then got smart and hired someone to do it for me. By 1990, I finally had enough of apartment living in New York City and bought a house in Port Jefferson, Long Island, on the North Shore. I transferred my college credits to the State University of New York at Stony Brook, and gladly made the switch to suburban life. I had a home of my very own and a familiar life of friendly neighbors, back yard barbeques, grass between my toes, and the sound of crickets to lull me to sleep at night. Long Island had plenty of beaches, boating, the sophistication of the Hamptons, and several world-class wineries. By car, I was about an hour to the city where I still had some business and three hours to upstate Newburgh. I felt like I had achieved the best of all possible worlds.

In only a few years, I accumulated a spectrum of knowledge in real estate and decided to try my luck as an independent real estate broker. I was far removed from the days when I thought Fannie Mae and her brother, Freddie Mac, were kindly old folks on some Southern front porch swing who gave money to needy people for home mortgages. I obtained a broker's license and focused on selling properties in the area where I lived. I took fewer than twenty clients at a time and worked non-stop; weekends, holidays, snowstorms; it didn't matter, as long as there was a sale to be made. One summer, my little 21-foot speedboat never saw water and sat on a trailer in my back yard.

In the early 1990s, the real estate market on Long Island was a bottomed-out nightmare for sellers and brokers like me. The national economy was precarious, mortgage rates fluctuated, and on Long Island, there were too many houses for sale and not enough qualified buyers. Customer service wasn't just a catchall word for me; it was the cornerstone of my business. I could've easily had a hundred clients and millions of dollars in gross inventory just like my competition, but like them, I would've failed to service the customer's needs. Being a successful real estate broker required more than just sticking a sign on the front lawn. It meant continuous knowledge of the community as well as changes in real estate law; it meant endless drive searches for homes to list, buy, or sell, as well as constant phone calls and networking. As the economy got worse, creative savvy and unconventional approaches were needed in order to survive as a business owner in the Long Island real estate market.

I worked from the convenient and more personable atmosphere of my home and served coffee to my clients at my kitchen table as we discussed their real estate needs. I took the time to understand and develop trust with my clients in an atmosphere devoid of corporate red tape or the intimidation of impressive suits, marble conference tables, and a display wall of framed honors. My commission was no less than the other brokers, but from me they'd receive frankness and a level of unpretentious service they'd find nowhere else. I returned phone calls. I knew the names of their kids, pets, and even watered their garden if they were away for the weekend. I did what ever it took to close the deal.

On one occasion, a minor crack on a toilet seat threatened to ruin my sale. The buyer refused to set a closing date unless the seller replaced it. Back and forth I talked to each party on the phone to negotiate a resolution. The adamant seller refused to replace the toilet seat and defended his home like a bear by saying that he'd, "…used that same toilet seat every day for thirty years and if it was good enough for him, it was good enough for them, too."

The idea of him seated at a toilet seat just wasn't the best visual response to convey back to the buyers from Staten Island, especially when it had taken me a year to get a sales contract for his home. He'd been with two other real estate agencies before me and now he was about to ruin everything. So, off to the hardware store I went to buy a new toilet seat. I installed it myself and for less than $20, the problem was settled and the house was sold.

The toilet seat episode, as it came to be known, helped to put things into perspective for me. By this time I was long overdue for a break and hadn't taken a vacation in years. I longed for new experiences beyond my work and just for a while, I needed to be in a place where I could hear my own thoughts again and where the daily grind of capitalism didn't consume my every waking moment and suck the life out of me. I'd always been inspired by the ancient history of Mediterranean cultures so I arranged for my business affairs to be managed and once every last detail was in order, I went to Greece for two months. I put my Porsche in the garage, threw some clothes in a backpack, and hired a limo to take me to Kennedy Airport. My only agenda was that I'd land in Athens the next morning.

In the first three weeks of the trip, I constantly called New York to check on my affairs. I was insane with guilt, couldn't relax and almost went home. Finally, I settled into the idea of a real vacation and decompressed. I couldn't believe I was in Greece. It was a place I had only seen in books and now I walked the same marble streets of great thinkers like Plato and Aristotle. A tremendous energy force still emanated from the ruins of magnificent ancient structures. My senses flooded with new experiences: museums held historic treasures, honeysuckle scented alleyways, freshly baked bread lured me, and an endless array of nightlife provided much needed fun.

After a week in Athens, I decided to head south to the Greek islands of Mykonos, Santorini, Ios, Serifos, and Paros. Each island had its own character and was speckled with even more archeological sites that filled my days with exploration and made me marvel at greatness gone by. I'd visit each island for a couple days before I hopped onto the next ship bound for some other Greek island.

I decided to go to the island of Icaria where the ancient myth says that Icarus, with his waxen wings, flew too close to the sun and fell into the sea. I'd forgotten the moral of that story and figured that poor foresight was the cause of his doom. Unlike the other islands I visited, the tourist map said that Icaria was a remote, rugged, mountainous island that few tourists visited. In tourist lingo, that meant it was cheap. Plus, it was only a three-hour trip by boat, which was soon to leave, so I boarded.

Starting out for the island of Icaria the weather was perfect. I handed the boatman my drachmas, which were the equivalent of about $2.00 and grabbed one of the few seats that remained, only a short distance from the helm. On previous island hops, I traveled on large ships with luxury accommodations, or on speed vessels called a Flying Dolphin; which were like a Lear Jet on water and were more expensive than the other passenger ships. By comparison, this trip to Icaria was taken in what I can only refer to as a large wooden fishing boat.

Its capacity was no more than fifty people, but more than twice that number filled the boat. The crew consisted of two men and there were no lifeboats, visible life preservers, or maximum occupancy signs anywhere. The captain was the very picture of a life-long seafarer with a weathered complexion, a scrabbled white beard, and strong arms. The boat had a small upper deck and the sides of the main deck were open and canopied. Most of the passengers made the best of the accommodations and went to the upper and rear decks in anticipation of a leisurely Mediterranean boat ride on a sunny afternoon.

I sat next to a British woman who traveled solo. She worked for British television and we continued to strike up friendly conversation as the boat motored away from the safety of the harbor and out to open sea. Suddenly, the waters churned, the winds grew wild and we found ourselves riding merciless swells to heights so great that only the blue sky could be seen until we'd crash back down with incredible force to meet the next swell. The vessel trembled against the forces as though it would break apart at any second.

The engine revved. Salt water and diesel fumes burned my eyes and fear settled on every face. The captain held the wheel with both hands as his first mate radioed the Greek Coast Guard to give our position. Wave after wave pounded the boat and we continued to ride great walls of water. The captain tried to take some swells from the side of the boat instead of head-on and barked out furious orders to his first mate. The two men spoke the quick and decisive language of peril and I could no longer translate, though the curse words they shouted in Greek were understood. They lit one cigarette after another and made the sign of the holy cross against their chests on numerous occasions, which drove my terror and made me swear like a sailor for my $2 decision.

Each time the boat groaned and shook, I wondered how my family would ever know the story of my death. My British friend and I were too stricken with fear to cry and expected at any moment to be tossed into the sea. Wet and shaken from the salty spray, we discussed how we might fare if that were to be the case and agreed that the odds weren't in our favor. Passengers who'd been on the upper deck now hovered for safety inside on the main deck. The poles, railings, and the backs of chairs bolted to the floor were their only means of support. Some passengers had only each other and their baggage to clutch onto. A young man of about twenty years old prayed loudly in Hebrew and each time the sea forced its way into the boat, people wailed with terror, and vomit swam across the floor.

LAND! The island of Icaria was in sight. Its great mountains rose up like a hostile giant and the jagged cliffs and jutting rocks along the coast posed new dangers as the sea threw our boat closer to the prospect of demise. The captain slammed the wheel to the left, fought his way around each boulder, and we slowly made our way into the harbor. Then, as if by some mercy of Poseidon, not only were we all alive, but the sea was peaceful again as though a great power switch had been turned off.

Six hours later we reached the dock, where an immense bronze statue of Icarus stood in the harbor. I could hardly wait to step onto land. Once tied to the dock, the Greek Coast Guard stepped on board. A feeling of "uh-oh" loomed and the captain of the boat was read the riot act for numerous violations. Traumatized, we all quickly exited. My legs trembled and the extra weight of my backpack didn't help to convince me that I stood on firm ground. It took three days for me to fully recover from that boat trip.

It was now close to sunset and my next goal was to find a cheap room with hot water and a private bathroom. The main village was within sight and at least a kilometer away. As I walked with my new British friend from the boat ride of doom, I offered to help her negotiate a room rate since I spoke some Greek and she didn't.

The stress of the day melted away as the sun warmed my face and the simplicity of island life was in full view. My friend and I trudged onward to the tourist village ahead as little children and dolphins played and swam in a clear blue harbor paradise. The warm breeze carried fresh scents of wild oregano from the mountainside; I breathed deeper for more. Outside a restaurant, freshly caught octopus hung on a line to soften in the sun and would be grilled to perfection that evening amid the sounds of bouzouki music, laughter, and the clanking sounds of beer mugs and bottles of Ouzo. Brightly colored houses welcomed me further, and narrow winding alleyways held friendly greetings from shopkeepers and passersby.

"Cali mera sas," said a man who walked by with his donkey in tow.

"Ya sas!" I replied. From a kitchen window, a mother called to her child. "Kostas! Ela dho!"

Finally, we came to an area of hotels and randomly went inside one to investigate further. A sixty-year-old woman greeted us. She was the owner of the small, family-owned hotel that had fifteen rooms for rent, each with a private bath, plenty of hot water and a balcony view of the sea. She'd make us a good deal if we both stayed five days. I translated the offer back into English for my British friend. The Greek woman then asked where we were from and I told her.

She looked surprised and confused at my reply and in her native tongue asked me, "Do you speak her language, too?"

"We speak the same language," I said. The woman looked perplexed.

"But how can you understand each other if she's from England

and you are American?"

I was baffled by the ignorance and innocence of her question, but concealed my disbelief so as not to offend her and explained that both countries spoke English. She still looked confused by this new piece of information but we continued to haggle in Greek for a low room rate. Experience taught me that I'd be out of business if I didn't know about my customers. Though I didn't ask, I wondered how she'd managed to escape knowledge of the English language when the majority of the world and her customer base consisted of foreign tourists. I later learned through conversations with her that she didn't own a television, had only an elementary level education, and hadn't left her island for more than thirty years when she attended her sister's wedding in Athens. Her insulated perspective of the world was contained on a tiny island in the Aegean Sea. We settled on a rate of $10 per room for five days and I looked forward to a soft pillow beneath my head.

In the years to come, I made other trips to Greece and saw incredible sights and met interesting people from all over the world, but I couldn't ever seem to shake off the memory of this one curious interaction. When the stress of work mounted and no relief was in sight, I'd think back to this one woman on a Greek island and wondered if ignorance was bliss. She didn't know about the outside world, didn't seem to care about it, or need to know, and that way of life worked for her. I wanted to explore the world and the people in it. I wanted to challenge, dissect, and push ideas to their very limits in order to understand and improve. I wondered whose view of life was better, hers, or mine. The question plagued me for years, but once being diagnosed with cancer, the answer was very clear to me; The brutal reality of truth is always preferable to the blossomed pain of ignorance.

The next day, my British friend and I set out for more adventure and rented an open jeep to explore the island. We woke up early, skipped breakfast, and tossed a few bottles of water in the back seat. Up the mountain we drove on the only paved road and soon found ourselves on rugged dirt trails that the map failed to reveal. We took turns driving the rutted, coastal route and maneuvered our way around large rocks and endless herds of goats. Soon, we were lost and a few times found ourselves on a cliff edge where the road had detoured or abruptly ended and the map failed to indicate any change. With teamwork and humor we found our way through each obstacle and at one point, gave up on the worthless map, agreed that we were totally lost, and now only relied on our instincts and hunger as a compass. No billboards, communication towers, or convenience stores existed, nor did any road signs. Whenever the road forked, or worse, came to a four-way intersection, we paused to weigh our decision, but wouldn't venture beyond the visibility of the coastline.

The air grew cooler as we climbed, but the intense Mediterranean sun still poured down on the flat-topped roofs of tiny village homes, which held layers of harvested figs, tomatoes, and olives to be dried for winter, as it had been done for generations. As the time of the siesta neared, we were famished. The siesta is a traditional part of the daily life of Mediterranean cultures where all work stops and businesses close from 1:00 – 4:00 p.m. The heat of the day is at its greatest during this time and people return to their homes to cook lunch, rest and re-connect with family. I had enormous difficulty with this concept at first and on a few occasions, found myself stomping my feet in public like a frustrated five-year-old because I was unable to exchange money, find a taxi, or even buy a stick of gum for hours. So, if we didn't stop to find food, we'd have nothing to eat. Except for the fact that we were on an island in the Greek Aegean, we didn't know where we were and were far away from any tourist location.

We arrived at a typical Greek village nestled in the side of a cliff, which was built over a millennium ago in a labyrinth style designed to confuse pirates and other marauders from nearby places like Morocco or Turkey who attacked and pillaged the inhabitants. The Icarian village consisted of about fifty whitewashed homes, a church, school, and a café, which also served as a post office and the town's main cultural and communication center. My friend and I entered the smoke-filled café where traditionally, respectable women unaccompanied by their men-folk are not permitted and are otherwise considered scandalous. We looked like a tumbled mess that blew into town. We were hungry, lost foreigners who wore tight blue jeans instead of skirts down to our ankles, and were caked with dust from the road. It helped that I spoke some Greek, which was an immediate icebreaker and their caution soon drifted to friendly conversation.

We bought them several shots of Ouzo as we filled our table with food and invited them to join us. Feta cheese, probably made from the goats we met along the road, as well as thick fresh bread, olives, stuffed grape leaves, and pasticcio was all that the café had to serve that day. We were grateful for every morsel. We were their entertainment and answered all of their curious questions. They couldn't understand why Americans bathed so much. Water, and hot water at that, was a scarce commodity throughout Greece. They figured that either Americans must be rich to take a shower every day, or were very dirty.

They were intrigued to know if we all drove a Buick and if everyone had a telephone and television in their home. There were many cars to choose from I told them and learned that a Camaro was the ultimate dream car of a few Icarian men. As for the telephone and television, I explained that not only did even the poorest Americans have them, but it was common to have more than one as I did. I was amazed to learn that this everyday fact in my experience, to them was too unbelievable. The very idea brought them to knee-slapping laughter as they wondered why anyone would want, or need more than just one television or phone. They roared with laughter and thought that I merely joked when I told them that some people had a phone in the bathroom. They were a simple people who lived off the land, took only what they needed, and didn't live to impress their neighbors. They traveled mostly by foot, donkey, or small fishing boat, were as rugged as the island they inhabited and full of dignity and pride for their culture.

They wanted to know what I thought of their island. I kept my complaints about the roads to myself. Their dialects were thick and I was slow to put sentences together. I apologized profusely for my lack, but they were patient, delightful, and flattered that a foreigner would even care to know their language and visit their village. Our hunger was now satisfied, but our bones ached from being jostled around in a jeep and we were ready to return to the tourist town. I fueled myself for the trip back with a double espresso and asked for directions, which played out like a village game of charades and provided us all with even more laughter.

Eventually, we found our way back down the mountain. After a long shower and a nap, I walked into town and spotted my British friend seated at a long table with a group of others at the local café. She waved me over and introduced me to a few people as everyone talked over plans for the evening. The sun cast brilliant colors as it set and the calm sea lightly ebbed. I wasn't sure if I wanted to do anything that evening except rest. The jeep tour and the boat ride from hell had me feeling overloaded, but I decided to sit for a while and enjoy a few stories and laughs over a cool drink beside the sea. Beer bottles clanked and fun conversation was heard all around. The group consisted of a dozen or so tourists, mostly Germans, some English, two French, one very angry Dutchman, and me, the only American. From the other side of the table I heard a voice of indignant surprise.

"She's American?" A tall, lanky man in his mid to late twenties, stood up, pointed at me like he'd just discovered a snake in Eden and asked, "Are you an American?" He looked as though he wanted to lunge at me, but I was at the opposite end of a crowded table with no room for him to maneuver. He spoke as though the word "American" was poison in his mouth. I was in no mood to be polite and didn't care to know the reason for his hostility.

"Yeah, I'm American. What of it?" I asked. "You got a problem with that?"

His eyes grew wide, his hands shook, and then, he erupted. He proceeded to rant about American military and foreign policy and said that we were all a bunch of back yard bullies who thought we owned the world. I took incredible offense at his words, but refused to make it obvious, or debate a fool. I thought of my family members who risked their lives and sacrificed personal freedoms in U.S. military service so that less fortunate people in the world could have justice, food, clothing, medicine, and weaponry enough to avoid being the victims of genocide. My fists clenched and my stomach knotted as he continued to degrade the land that I love.

With every sentence he strove to make a mockery of American values and democracy. I now wished he were at my end of the table so that he'd swallow his teeth with one blow of my fist. My British friend and I continued to talk about plans for the evening and attempted to ignore him as he attempted to incite me into political debate and attacked everything American. Mostly, I laughed at him, which turned him bright red and at one point I said, "Hey, man, this isn't the United Nations. I'm on vacation, so go protest somewhere else. If you don't like America then write a letter to the President. Shut up, and don't bother me with your stupid problems." At that, the German side of the table gasped with shock, one lady shifted her eyes downward, and even the French seemed a little unsettled. Somehow I'd crossed an invisible line but didn't know how. Then, someone nearby told me that "shut up" was the equivalent of the four-lettered F-word that many Americans use frequently but sophisticated Europeans did not. Even in the worst of verbal confrontations, a mere "shut up" by their standards was excessive force and was like a machete whack across the knees. I didn't care about their definitions and made no apologies whatsoever. I was pleased that I'd managed a double-dog dare and now the Dutchman had to either make a comeback or shut up for good. The others seated at the table were silent, and lit shaky cigarettes in anticipation of the next step of this ridiculous face-off. The Dutchman still stood at the end of the table and finally, one person grabbed his arm and told him to sit down.

"Hey, she's just a woman," the man said, but the angry Dutchman wouldn't stop.

To him, I was an American to be berated, humiliated, and publicly flogged for offenses dating back to before the Civil War. His next and last attempt to be victorious was a weak one. Unable to corner me on the ropes of a political debate, he settled for schoolyard tactics. "You Americans are all narrow-minded. What do you know about any other country, but your own? Pick one country, just pick one," he challenged.

Ah! I thought as I sensed the approach of an easier game and got ready to dangle his stupidity over his own hot flame. "Okay," I said, "how about your country?"

He sneered, "Holland? What do you know about Holland?"

The fact that ancestors from my maternal grandmother's side came to America from Holland seemed a moot point to share with him. I also came from French, Sicilian, English, Irish, and Canadian Indian lineage but none of that worldliness seemed appropriate to share either. I could have walked away from the Dutchman at any point, but if I did, he would've won by default. So, I stayed just to show him that he had no authority and enjoyed the fact that he was so irritated by my presence.

"Let me see how smart you are, you American," he taunted. "I'll bet you can't name three things about Holland. Go ahead; see if you can do it. Just name three things about Holland." He held up three fingers as if I needed a visual confirmation of the number three and then stood with his arms folded as though he held court. I entered this battle without patience, now had even less, and was ready to give a pie in the face answer to end it once and for all.

"Well, let me see," I said, "three things about Holland," and pretended to think really hard. "I've got it," I said. "You haven't given anything new to the world since tulips and windmills, you wear wooden shoes, and you're all a bunch of prostitutes and heroine addicts. There," I said, "that's more than three!"

The table exploded with laughter and the Dutchman stormed off. I never saw him again, but that one situation by the Mediterranean Sea was a lesson that I never forgot: Enemies strike when you least expect it, but the element of surprise doesn't necessarily equal defeat. Readiness to defend will always be required, unconventional tactics might be best, and at the very least, even bad humor is a weapon.

***

Maureen called me one day with great news. She was engaged! I'd recently returned from another trip to Greece and wanted to catch up on all the news with her.

"Hey," I said, "one of my clients gave me tickets to a Mets game this Friday at Shea Stadium. Let's go and we'll talk about everything."

"You don't even like baseball," she reminded me. Maureen loved baseball. Her father loved baseball. Even my Grandmother Miller was a huge Yankees fan, but somehow, I never sat still long enough to learn about it.

As we watched the game, Maureen and I talked about her wedding scheduled for the following fall of 1994. It would be one of the most spectacular weddings I ever attended. A U.S. citizen for more than a decade, her fiancé Barry was from Ireland. A plane full of his family and friends from the land of luck flew to New York to join them in celebration and a blessing from the Vatican was read in the cathedral.

But still a year away, Maureen already had many wedding details in order. Her gown would be silk with a row of buttons down the back. There'd be ice sculptures, a white horse-drawn carriage, a live Irish band, lavish food, and miniature bottles of Bailey's Irish Crème at each place setting. She was thrilled about the future. Suddenly, the stadium roared and Maureen cheered.

"What happened?" I asked.

"You didn't see that? It was a triple play," she said with excitement.

"What's a triple play?" I asked.

"Oh, brother!" Maureen rolled her eyes and shook her head in disbelief. With her hand on her hip she playfully teased, "That's right! What would a prissy, high school basketball cheerleader know about America's favorite pastime?"

We laughed as we remembered our high school days. Ten years earlier, I had pranced around the gym at Wallkill High School with bells on my shoes, did splits and cartwheels, all while Maureen slugged baseballs out of the field for the varsity team.

***

Maureen was pregnant soon after her honeymoon. Her baby shower came and went and her August due date approached on schedule. She called me from her hospital bed, "The baby is doing great. It's a boy. He's perfect and I have cancer."

I was speechless. She explained that the delivery moved along normally until at one point she struggled to breathe. The doctors put her on oxygen and afterward, tests found that a cancerous tumor was wrapped around her heart. Maureen had Non-Hodgkin's Lymphoma and immediately began chemotherapy. Her doctor later explained that cancer symptoms can be masked by pregnancy and elevated hormones can even increase cancer cell growth. It was all too great a shock. How could Maureen have a healthy new baby and cancer, too? The injustice was enormous.

"I'm going to beat this, you'll see," she said to me one day when I visited. No one ever doubted for a moment that she would. If anyone could beat cancer, it was Maureen. She had everything to live for and was one of the most fearless people I knew. Maureen was even proud of her bald appearance and made no efforts to conceal it.

At the time of her illness, my life was in high turmoil and turnover. I felt uncertain about my career, future, how I fit into the world, and felt unable to support Maureen during her worst time. Since my first trip to Greece, I'd seriously considered the need for a life overhaul but continued to get caught up in the day-to-day of business. There was always one more deal and I could never seem to make a clean break to start over. My love life was in the crapper too and at twenty-nine years old, prospects for a happy, life-long marriage with someone seemed slim to none from my vantage point anyway. In general, I'd grown too picky about my likes and dislikes and this carried over into my non-existent romantic life.

In my dating life, my criteria were extensive. I was overly cautious and my tolerance level was too short. I'd reached the point of no return and was unwilling to waste my time on thirty-something men who didn't know how to treat a lady, were non-committal, and didn't even know what they wanted out of life. So, I drew a line in the sand and conducted many dates more like a cross-examination, or job interview with few second interviews being granted. Dating and romance was supposed to be fun, but I wasn't having fun at all. I wanted to be married and have a family, but wouldn't compromise my values or integrity. One day I phoned Maureen to talk about it all just like we had always done with each other since we were teenagers.

"So what's happening? How are you?" she asked me. She had a chemo treatment earlier that day and periodically the conversation broke as she dry heaved. She'd groan from exhaustion, and then apologize.

"Maureen, don't apologize for being sick," I said. "Maybe this isn't such a good time to talk."

"No. No. That's okay," she insisted. She was determined to chat on the phone like the old days and not let her illness interfere. As I continued to complain about my life, I could hear her baby cry in the background.

"Do you want to trade places?" she asked me.

I felt like an insensitive jerk. The strange fact was that I had cancer too. I just didn't know it yet.

"Don't go out with that guy anymore," she scolded me, "he's a loser. Dump him. You have to find someone like my Barry, who loves you no matter what."

How in the world I'd find a guy like that I didn't know. I never went out anymore and when I wasn't at work, I had my face in a book for college. Unless the perfect man fell from the sky and landed at my feet cloaked in flashing neon red to make me take notice, it was unlikely that I'd ever find my dream man.

A year later, a lot had changed for me. Business on Long Island was at its worst in 1996 and home sales plummeted even lower. I took myself out of the real estate game. I was tired of the struggle, was overburdened, and suffocated with responsibilities for far too long. I just couldn't imagine another ten years of the same old thing and needed my life to be a lot easier, if only for a while. I wanted to finish the bachelor's degree that I'd started more than a decade earlier and just wanted to think, breathe for a while, and regroup.

My rental properties were sold as well as the antique, mahogany baby grand piano with ivory keys that I scooped for $100 at a yard sale. I sold my house and the boat in the back yard was practically given away. I happily purged my old way of life and got rid of many material trophies which had outwardly been a measure of my success by societal standards, but inwardly, never meant that much to me at all. It was now all a burden and slowed me down in my quest for peace of mind. My Greek travels taught me how to live free and that meant fewer possessions.

So, with no angst whatsoever, I sold the Porsche. It was a happy day when I handed the keys to its new owner. For one reason or another that car was a headache and cost twice as much for a simple oil change than my ten-year-old Dodge Daytona. I kept the Dodge. It had high miles but was hardly a clunker. It gave me no problems and with one turn of the key, never failed to start on the coldest winter days. One day, in my new studio apartment, I prayed about it all and included the wish for my dream man to arrive soon or else I was willing to be single forever.

"Now God," I pleaded, "I know I'm picky, but it's really important that he understand that I won't change my last name. I just won't do it, God."

Okay, okay, everyone has a quirk and that one was mine. Probably as a result of too many Victorian literature and sociology courses, it had long been my rebellious contention that I was not chattel to be exchanged between men, and to the woe of my family, I refused to change, or even hyphenate my name for the purpose of marriage. Few men that I dated ever agreed to this and those that did, I didn't believe anyway.

By this time, I was jobless, it was holiday time, and I needed the security of a weekly paycheck. I told the lady at the employment agency, "Just get me a job that I don't have to think about after 5 o' clock, or on weekends."

On the first day of December, I reported to my new job as Administrative Assistant to the Vice President of Customer Service. Two friendly women came by my desk and introduced themselves and before I knew it, the "get to know you" transitioned into an inquiry about the status of my love life. "Love was in the water" at this company, the two women told me. Several co-workers not only dated, but a few even married and they whipped out pictures to show me.

"Oh," I said, "I have a policy; I don't date the men that I work with."

They were undeterred in their matchmaking pursuits and continued to describe several available bachelors. I gave a disinterested snub to each for one reason or another.

"I know who's perfect for you," said the one, and proceeded to rave about a kind-hearted, fun-loving, laid-back guy in the Information Technology department. The other woman agreed and together their eyes twinkled with possibilities.

"Hmmm," I said with half interest, "what's his name?" Heck, I didn't even have a name badge or computer yet - I was just making chitchat with these ladies as they stood at my desk.

"Joey Miller," they said.

"Miller? His last name is Miller? My last name is Miller," I said.

They couldn't believe it and we laughed.

"Can you imagine if you two get married?" said one woman. "You wouldn't have to change your name!"

"Yeah, but he's probably like all the rest of the single guys. They're all the same."

"Oh, no", said one, "not Joey, I've known him for five years. He's a keeper."

"So, how come you don't date him if he's so wonderful?" I asked.

"Joey? He's like a brother." They both nodded.

"Great," I chimed, "just who I want to date, my brother!" I don't know why, but I continued to ask questions about this mystery man and they shared all kinds of stories, including one when he sent Valentine's Day flowers to all the single women in the office with no boyfriend. That's when I started to be a little interested.

"C'mon, you've got to meet him," they said and before I knew it I was being led down the hallways to the other side of the building to meet some strange man named Joey Miller.

"What's the game plan?" I asked as the three of us first fluffed up our hair and checked our make-up. "What am I supposed to say? "Hi, I have the same last name as you?"

"We'll just be nonchalant like we're giving you a tour of the building on your first day. If sparks fly, then they fly. If not, then no big deal," they told me. Like thirteen-year-olds, the three of us giggled in anticipation all the way and by the time we got to Joey's office, it didn't take a genius to figure out what we were up to.

There he was. Joey Miller. My first impression was that he looked like a great thinker, a scientist type with a close-cropped beard, and glasses. I was cautiously interested. What I didn't know was that he was already interested in me. A month earlier, he'd given me a flirtatious "hello" as he passed by me in the hallway on the day of my interview, but I didn't remember him. With my new matchmaking office pals, we stood in front of Joey with stupid grins and giggles as he asked what we were up to, which made us giggle some more. He gave us a quizzical look. The two women blushed with guilty transparency. Sparks flew between Joey and me, but were slow to light the sky.

Two weeks later I had plans to meet friends in Manhattan for a holiday party and would catch a train into Penn Station right after work. It snowed that afternoon and ice covered the parking lot. My Dodge Daytona wouldn't start. It had never happened before. Joey offered to drive me to the train station and I accepted. We stood together on the platform and waited for the train to arrive. The temperature was unbearably frigid and my teeth chattered. I forgot my gloves so he gave me his. He was leaving the next day to fly to Indiana for the holidays and would be back in two weeks. We talked about the possibility of dinner and a movie when he got back. He kept the offer casual, like it wasn't really a date, but I could see that he was interested and I was too.

Finally, the train arrived and the heat from the tracks mixed with the cold air and created a foggy mist like some romantic black and white movie from the 1940s. As we said our goodbyes, and wished each other a happy holiday, a magnetic linger was present between us. I boarded, waved and watched him walk away as the mist from the tracks wafted up around him. I'd be in Manhattan in an hour to dance and laugh the night way, but as I sat on the train, all I could think about was Joey Miller. A week later he called me from his parents' house in Indiana to say that he'd been thinking of me too. I had butterflies in my stomach, but was still a little cautious. On his return, he asked me on several dates, but I made lame excuses each time: I had an aerobics class, an Italian class, and even once said that I couldn't go out with him because I had to wash my hair.

Up to this point, Joey and I had made polite conversation here and there, but shyness and a need to maintain professionalism prevented more than that. Finally, I realized that if I didn't at least go on one date with him, he'd stop asking, so by the end of January, I agreed to go to dinner after work. The loud silence at our table was awkward at first, but then he asked me, "So what do you want out of life?"

It was on. I laid it all on the table like a well-rehearsed presentation with charts, graphs, and spreadsheets.

"Look," I said, "I know this is totally against the first date rules, but I'm not about to pretend and waste five years trying to figure out if you want the same thing out of life as I do. At the very worst, we'll have a nice dinner and still say hello to each other in the hallways at work." He appreciated my boldness and also wanted the same: marriage, family, a nice home, and a good job. It all seemed very simple, but for some reason both of us hadn't struck the lottery yet in the love department. We liked each other, but being on the cautious side, decided to keep things casual and for months, most of our co-workers didn't even know that we dated.

After about seven months of dating, it was clear that Joey and I liked each other a great deal, but on his part, I wasn't sure to what extent. As for myself, my feelings became clearer to me one morning as I drove to work. I spotted Joey's car only a few cars ahead of mine and decided to inch my way up in the hope of getting behind him to surprise him with a beep and a wave. Finally, I made my way through traffic and when I got behind his car and saw the back of his head all I could manage was this thought; Gee, I could marry that man. A couple of months later, I knew how Joey really felt about me when he handed me a present. Inside a pretty papered box, no bigger than the size of my palm was a glass, heart-shaped jewelry box.

"It's my heart," he said, "and it belongs to you."

***

During the late summer and early autumn of 1997, Joey traveled back and forth to a client in Dallas, Texas. Every week for months, I picked him up at LaGuardia Airport late on Friday nights. On Saturday, we barely had time to catch up with each other in between the laundry and re-packing for his flight back to Texas. On Sunday, we'd grab breakfast at the local diner and visit on the drive to the airport. Always, Joey excitedly talked about Texas and wanted me to visit Dallas for a weekend, but I made excuses every time. I didn't want to visit Dallas and figured that aside from the infamous grassy knoll, and a bunch of steak joints, there was nothing to see. Joey told me about great nightlife comparable to New York as well as art museums, several nearby universities, friendly people, an economy that boomed with opportunities, and yes, there was even sushi. He brought back lots of real estate magazines for me to peruse and it all sounded too good to be true.

"Anyway," I said, "who wants to go to a place with tumbleweeds in the streets and cactus everywhere? Doesn't everyone still ride horses in Texas? I'll bet there aren't any shopping malls."

Joey described further the realities of North Texas in near 21st century. There were trees, not cactus. He hadn't seen any tumbleweed. People drove cars and very nice ones too and there were beautiful homes for half the price of what it cost in New York, as well as Gallerias enough to please even a 5th Avenue shopper. I couldn't believe it and was shocked to know that such a life existed outside New York and for far less money. But Joey had lived in Chicago, Miami, and San Francisco prior to moving to New York and knew better. He'd lived in New York about five years before we met, didn't like it at all and told me many times his long list of reasons, which I knew to be true, but figured that's just the way life was. I hadn't ever considered a life outside of New York and had no reason to give it serious thought. So, I didn't.

On one of Joey's weekend trips back to New York, we walked on the pier in downtown Port Jefferson and talked about the company in Dallas.

"They'd be smart if they hired me with all the money they spend on my plane tickets every week," he said with a mixture of seriousness and humor.

"Yeah right," I laughed and figured that would happen when hell froze over and pigs flew. He liked the people at the company in Plano and they liked and trusted his ability. About four months later, he was offered a job, which prompted pivotal decisions in our relationship. The job market was awful in New York and had been for a long while with no relief in sight. We'd even talked about getting an apartment together closer to the city where jobs were in higher volume. I didn't want to live in any one of the five New York City boroughs ever again, nor did I want Joey to endure the stress of Long Island commuter trains every day to Manhattan.

Where once I never dreamed of leaving New York, now I knew that it was the best thing for Joey and there were no more decisions to be made. I'd go with him and take my chances on a place that I knew only from cowboy movies. We moved to Texas in April 1998, were engaged that December and the next year, built a new house in the city of Allen before we married in 2000. And that's how this New York girl made her way to Texas.

***

Except for two suitcases of clothes, we packed up everything, Joey's car included, on a moving van that would drive down the East Coast and meet up with us in Texas in two weeks. I sold my Dodge Daytona for a dollar to a co-worker in desperate need of a vehicle. Before leaving for Texas I received word that Maureen had died after an attempt at one more research drug. It was a strange feeling to know that my friend was dead while I flew to the promise of a new life with the man I loved. I had no idea that a cancerous tumor sat with us in first class as we sipped champagne and toasted our future.

A few hours later we arrived in Dallas. My first impressions of Texas were made in the car on the way out of the airport. I'd never seen so much development in my life: highways, big buildings, and real estate signs were everywhere. The newness thrilled me. Until the truck with all of our possessions arrived, we lived out of suitcases in a hotel and ate at restaurants until we found an apartment. After we got situated at the hotel, we went to a popular restaurant chain for dinner and on my first night in Texas I got more than just a huge portion of food. Aside from all the miles of growth and expansion, I was also struck by how friendly people were, and for no apparent reason.

"So how y'all doin' tonight?" our waiter asked. He was young, enthusiastic and took a seat right next to me in our booth as if he had done it a hundred times before. His immediate familiarity alarmed me and caution flares ignited in every brain cell as I clutched my purse closer to my body like a passenger on a New York subway.

"Y'all fixin' to go to a movie or something after dinner?" he asked with a singsong bounce and a smile. Still pensive, I moved my purse out of sight and didn't reply, but Joey returned friendly conversation as the waiter took our order and left to bring us our drinks.

"What's his problem?" I asked Joey.

"What do you mean?" Joey asked as if nothing was unusual.

"He sat next to me, that's what," I said. "I never had a waiter do that in my life and why does he want to know what we're 'doin' tonight? It's suspicious. What does he care?" I paused. "Do you think he's trying to get our guard down so that he can work some kind of con game on us?"

Joey looked at me like I was crazy. "Michelle, he's being friendly. People are nice here so get used to it. You're not in New York anymore."

"Oh," I said, and was a little embarrassed. Experience had been my teacher. The cutthroat, fast-paced business world proved that others not only perceived niceties as a weakness, but often times they carried ulterior motives too. Caution was a daily tactic and survival had to be learned quickly on the streets of New York City where unsolicited conversations with strangers that extended beyond, "Excuse me, do you have the time?" might equal trouble in the form of robbery, rape, or death. And though I'd been raised in the countryside of upstate New York, full of neighborliness and charitable good will, that side of my character wouldn't make a huge difference in the lives of others until my cancer diagnosis met with opportunity two years later, in Texas.

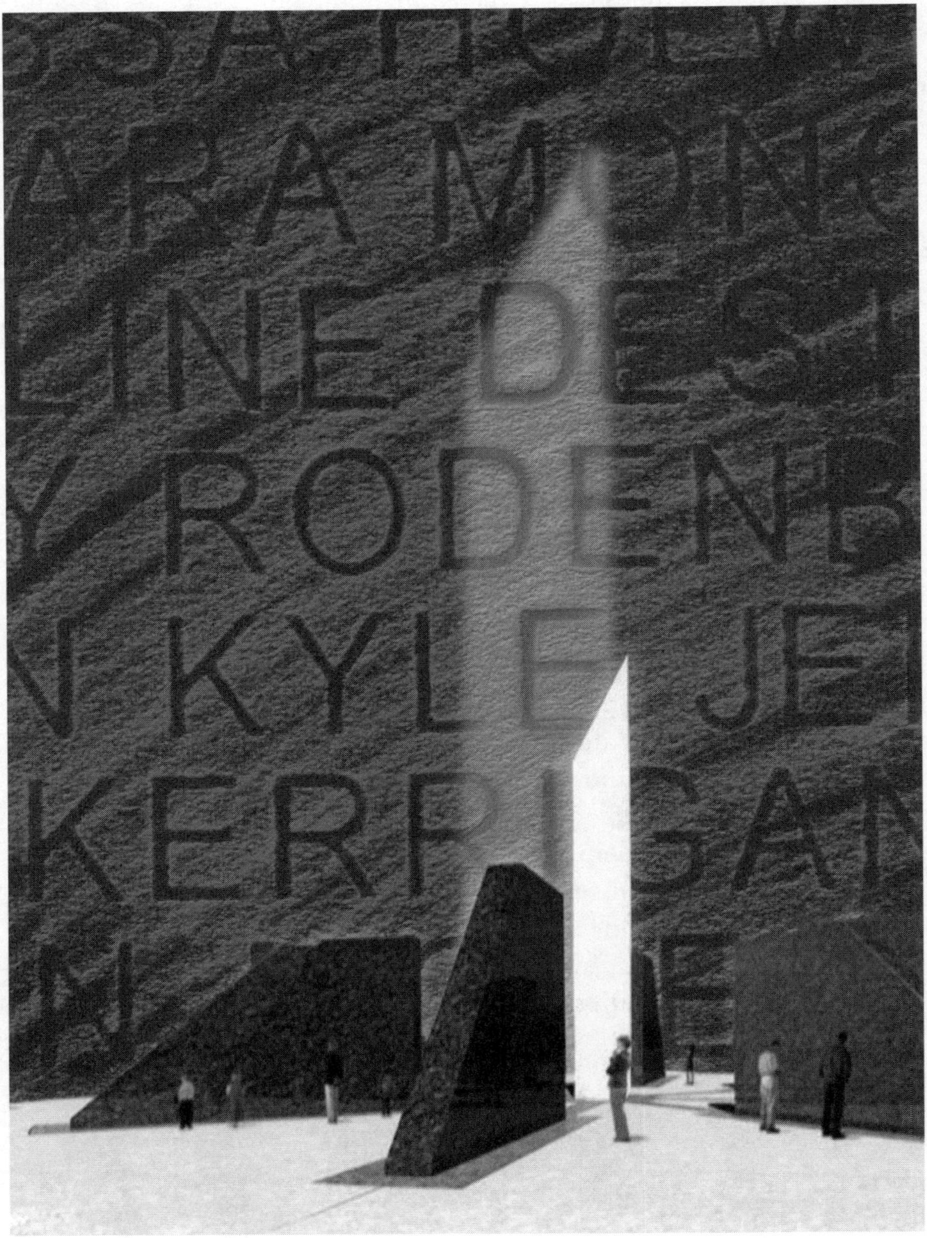

Graphic Composition by Annie Gough

Chapter 3
Locked and Loaded: The New Normal

Except for a few people, I didn't discuss the monument. I was content to quietly document what I'd envisioned that day in my living room. I organized concepts, planned short and long-term goals, and sketched the monument's design as best as my basic artistic talents allowed. I wasn't sure yet of the next step to take to get the monument built, but I knew that it would require the commitment of many people who cared as much as I did. In the meantime, I wrote poetry, kept a journal, read my favorite books, and when I wasn't working on The Cancer Monument, I learned as much as I could about cancer.

Nearly every day, cancer treatments brought routine hardships and some unexpected issues as well. One day I realized that my saliva tasted like a mouthful of pennies and no matter what I did, it didn't go away. I asked the nurse why this was so.

"Oh, that's normal," she said, "it's the destroyed iron in your blood. It'll flush out, just drink a lot of water."

While I was glad to know that the dead blood would flush out of my system, I was grossed out with this all too clear image of the voluntary, extensive, and routine damage being done to my body in order to become cancer-free. Some suggestions were made to help alleviate the metal taste: chocolate, peanut butter, gravy, and creamy sauces might help to make foods taste better but also helped to pack on extra pounds, which I didn't need. So, I preferred to taste metal instead. Until I was finished with chemo, foods like tuna fish, anything made from tomatoes, or citrus fruits now clashed with the taste in my mouth. I sought the advice of a nutritionist just to be sure that I ate right during this critical time when vitamins, minerals, and calories were of high importance.

On some days I lacked enough energy to open a can of soup much less prepare a nutritious meal, but I forced myself to eat from the five food groups, drink plenty of water, and take a multi vitamin to help repair damage and refuel for the battle ahead. Before chemotherapy, once a meal was chewed and swallowed, I never stopped to consider the process, but just a few months into chemo, I was forced to rethink the whole thing, make adjustments, eat smaller meals, or deal with the consequences of extreme fatigue. The effort to prepare a meal, eat it and digest was now equated with bodily work that required a great deal of energy from my already weakened body.

Ordinarily, digestion requires a great amount of blood, enzymes and stomach acids, which work to break down foods and deliver nutrients to cells. I now lacked normal levels of digestive agents, including healthy red blood cells due to chemo. The blood sent to my stomach to digest a simple meal resulted in a total energy deficit and had the power to weaken, make me dizzy, and took me off my feet for several hours. A steak dinner, or heavy Italian meals were now off limits. Unless I ate light meals with easily digestible proteins, I could be glassy-eyed with little energy to even hold up my head, or make intelligent conversation without slurred speech. When my white cells were low and caused me to be susceptible to infection, my favorite food, sushi, was off limits. A bout with food poisoning probably would have killed me, and for once, I didn't tempt fate.

My chemotherapy sessions were every two weeks and just as my body started to recover, I'd be hit again with a heavy dose of poison. I started to feel like a little flower watered with bleach when all I wanted to do was just grow roots, bask in the dewy morning sunshine, and be free of weeds. Traditional chemo kills cancer cells, the doctors and nurses explained, but it can't distinguish a healthy cell from an unhealthy one, so millions of my healthy cells were destroyed too, which not only destroyed my blood, and weakened me, but also left me unable to fight off infection for weeks at a time. As a result, I was in a perpetual state of alert over ordinary germs and at times wondered what might kill me first, cancer treatments, or cancer itself. This, combined with many more uncertainties that I couldn't control, were at times difficult to cope with if I thought about them for too long. I had a life beyond cancer and refused to forego the other things that were important to me, like my marriage, education, and career.

My emotions sometimes swung like a pendulum, insomnia was a constant and everything compounded as a result of the steroids I was given with chemo. I'd have long periods of coping well and then on any given moment could be overtaken by some new situation that sparked new fears and frustrations. Anti-depressants would have been a fast fix but wouldn't get to the root of the problem. I wasn't the type to take anti-depressants anyway and believed that the ability to cope had to come from within me. Heck, I barely ever took an aspirin for a headache. I didn't want any more drugs in my body, but I was committed to the action plan made with my oncologist and had months of more chemo. More and more I recognized that my need to cope evolved, and soon enough I realized what I needed most - balance. Somehow, I'd have to strike a balance within the chaos in order to keep fully in life, and in pursuit of the goals that I planned for myself.

At times, I viewed my crisis as if it were a scale. One side of the scale had the weight of a cancer crisis and the other side was way up in the air. My job was to balance the scale and securely place the things that were important to me that had nothing to do with cancer on the other side. When people assumed that just living my life served as a distraction from my cancer it really irked me. You can't be distracted from cancer, but you can continue living. No matter how fun diversions may be, it's impossible to evade cancer if you have it. A purposeful life was my goal and I strove to find strategies and techniques to manage the everyday challenges of my illness so that I could thrive.

The more I thought about the topic of balance, I began to wonder if I'd ever had it. Sure, there were days, maybe even weeks or months that balance existed for me. But as a way of life, I'd been less than deliberate in this matter as I had been in others. Over a long period of time and for all of my assertiveness, I'd allowed my boundaries and long-term peace of mind to be bulldozed by various people and situations. This, combined with a host of other negative stresses like: toxic air, polluted water, foods grown in depleted soil, hormones in animals, mercury in fish, glues in carpeting, electric or radio wave currents from household appliances, chemicals in ordinary house paint, detergents, cleaning products, and a thousand other everyday pollutants have the potential effect of a nail in a tire. There are many risk factors that contribute to cancer, but many answers are still needed. Why it is that a forty-year smoker doesn't get cancer but a child does? This is one such question that science can't answer with certainty just yet. One bad cell can begin the regeneration of many millions into a cancerous tumor and until research can do more, we must protect ourselves from cancer as best as possible.

In the meantime, my main challenge is to live as a cancer survivor, to live with the side effects, as well as concerns about what may happen twenty years from now as a result of cancer therapies that I took. My quest is to make a quality life for myself whether with, or beyond, a cancer diagnosis. I'll never know what caused my cancer and I don't obsess over the past. Everyday, I make a conscious effort to live for the future.

So, once I recognized that I needed balance like never before, I had to learn how to assert, practice, and hold on to it as a new way of life no matter what. That was the hard part. No one mentioned to me the deep philosophical confusion that cancer would create: acceptance of inward and outward transformations, my societal worth, relationships with others, and purpose in life—it was all so much! If that weren't enough, from time to time I'd remember the nurse's words, "Chemo can burn a hole in your bladder, so be sure to urinate frequently," and then I'd worry about that possibility and drank tons of water every day just to help flush everything along. The smells that came out of me as a result of chemo drugs were freakishly unnatural. No one told me to expect that. It was hard to feel like a vibrant woman when alien chemicals putrefied my 'innards' and constipated me beyond the ability of over the counter laxatives.

I felt like I had a continuous hangover and my sense of smell heightened to the level of dogs and cats. Before Joey left for work each morning, he'd kiss me. His cologne and minty fresh breath within a two foot radius made me cringe, groan, and hold my hand out to stop him from coming any closer. He learned not to take such aversions personally. We made adjustments to our routine; he didn't wear cologne while I was in treatment and kissed me before he brushed his teeth. As chemo continued, the effort of standing was at times too great even just to take a shower; it could deplete me of energy so fast that I'd have to lay down for at least fifteen minutes before I continued. Still dripping wet and with enough energy to stagger to the bed and lay down, I'd rest for a bit, regain my energy, and then get dressed. Before I was ready to walk out the door, I was already exhausted. Except for Joey and a few close friends and family, most people never saw the great levels of unpredictable fatigue that were the result of cancer treatments. Instead, they saw a put-together person who burst with enough energy to laugh and talk with friends at lunch, a Foundation fundraiser, or a literature class. They didn't see that when I went home, I fell on the couch in an exhausted heap or that the next day I'd be bed ridden.

To help with the fatigue issues of daily showering, we bought a shower bench. Though I needed it, my pride kicked in for a couple of days anyway, I tried not to use it just to prove to myself that I was really okay. The shower bench made me super aware that I was sick, just like the day when my hair first fell out. But fatigue won out over my ego and I couldn't avoid the fact that I needed the bench. The loss of oxygenated red blood cells due to chemo also created shortness of breath, which made even the most ordinary conversations a physical feat and zapped me of energy so badly that sometimes I slurred my words as if I were drunk. My job required that I talk all day long and caused my lungs and throat to be so raw that I couldn't sleep at night. These once simple actions of conversation and laughter were now daily challenges.

In order to function, I began to think of my energy in economic terms. Bodily energy was now like money in the bank. If I borrowed too much in one area, I'd sacrifice another and if I used it all up without a careful plan, I'd be bankrupt. I began to practice this new philosophy and slowly worked towards a new rhythm and perspective for myself within the daily challenges of cancer. As a result, I became better at time management, learned to establish better boundaries with others, and strove towards much-needed balance.

Then, one day in late June, my chest ached and uncontrollable fever raged. When we arrived at the emergency room I was delirious and could barely keep my eyes open, but still had the presence of mind to insist on a private hospital room. The last thing I'd get at the hospital was privacy. For the first two days the doctors didn't know what the problem was, but kept me in ice packs and my veins full of antibiotics. The medical staff went in and out of my room all night to take vital signs.

The only times that I'd been admitted into a hospital was for my birth and a tonsillectomy when I was age two. I was frightened. My mother was a nurse for more than twenty-five years; I was scared from the hospital stories that I'd heard from her. In addition, the rare and horrible news stories about raped patients and negligent deaths furthered my worries. To exacerbate my concerns, I experienced the most ignorant and uncompassionate care I hope to ever endure. While in the emergency room, four different people, including a doctor, tried to access my medi-port a total of eleven times. Eleven times I was stabbed in the chest with a one-inch needle as I kicked and screamed in agony and Joey was nearby to watch it all. By this time, my fever was 103 degrees, it hurt just to keep my eyes open, I had no patience, and the profanity and threats that roared out of me reached record levels. As I lay on an examination table, I told everyone that if my port were accessed one more time they'd get my fist. That's the nice version of what I said. After getting into my hospital room, I still fumed over this incident but had clarity of mind to write a formal complaint and continued my protest to a hospital administrator. She was very apologetic and agreed that I had received poor treatment and also said that most emergency room personnel had no experience with medi-ports.

"So why the hell did they try eleven times?" I asked. She had no answer. In the years to come, I'd talk about this incident many times to nurses, doctors, and lab technicians, and especially as a warning to any newcomers whose responsibility it was to stick me with a needle. It was always the same; everyone was shocked at my one horrible E.R. experience. The experience damaged my already weakened trust for the medical profession and from then on, Joey and I never assumed that I'd receive excellent care. Instead, we made it our business to ask a lot of questions no matter how ignorant they appeared, got to know hospital staff workers, and with my oncology care team, we developed very close relationships.

Still with fever, I needed to be hooked to an I.V. so that I could receive antibiotics. I wouldn't let anyone touch me and then, the most wonderful I.V. nurse named Jenny entered the room. I'd never heard of an I.V. nurse before. In disbelief, Jenny listened to my horrible E.R. story and then she armed Joey and me with needed information that we use to this day.

"The next time you walk into this hospital or anywhere where you don't have your regular care team and your port needs to be accessed," she said, "you ask for me or if I'm not here, ask for anyone on the I.V. team. Don't let anyone else touch your port because chances are that they don't know how. Just ask for Jenny, everyone knows me here." I'd have to go to this hospital several more times for routine CT and Gallium scans and soon learned that everyone indeed knew Jenny by her first name only, like Cher, or Oprah. Jenny was definitely my super star that day.

From then on, if any needles came in close proximity, I'd say, "Can you please call Jenny?" My trust level climbed because of Jenny's bedside manner and most of all, for her interest to inform me. She treated me like a person instead of a disease and I felt more empowered as a result. But, before I'd let her stick me in the chest to access my port, I continued my little interview process to know her credentials and to also negotiate the terms for needle stick number twelve. At this point, my chest was raw around my heart where the port was located and combined with the previous eleven pokes, I now felt like road kill.

"One stick," Jenny promised. "I'll get it one stick. Just take a deep breath and hold it." I'd been in fight mode for about two hours by this time and had no more energy to debate Jenny, or the hospital administrator. One big and painful stick in the chest later the port was accessed. Antibiotics and narcotics flowed to relieve the pain that seared through my skull. My adrenaline pumped so hard that drugs did nothing to slow me down, much to the amazement of the nurses.

"She's still talking?" the nurse questioned in amazement.

"Yeah, she's pretty worked up," Joey said, "It's hard to stop her once that happens," he smiled.

After the nurses left the room, I turned to Joey and said, "Don't leave me. These people don't care about me." My eyes pleaded and he held my hand. Because of what I'd experienced in the E.R., my initial suspicions about being perceived as a worthless cancer victim were to me, less speculative, and now a reality of life threatening proportions. I thought, why would these total strangers care about me in the first place? In my state of crisis, I didn't stop to consider Hippocratic oaths taken, ongoing training, licenses, or the fact that the overwhelming majority of medical professionals cared. All I knew was that I fought for my life and wasn't about to freely give trust to anyone who just happened to be at the other end of my rope.

"What if they hurt me again, or what if I'm in a coma and can't speak for myself?" I asked Joey in desperation. "Who'll protect me if you're not here? Stay with me, please."

"I'm right here. I'm not leaving you, don't worry," Joey said.

For two days, we didn't know why fevers raged. In the meantime, I learned how to survive in the strangeness of the hospital environment. I refused to let my guard down, so I fought to stay awake against the strength of the narcotics. I wanted to be able to identify the face of every person who came into my room, even those who came at 3:00 a.m. for routine vital signs and to pack my body in more ice. It didn't take me long to realize how over-burdened the hospital staff was, the nurses especially. The pain of constant high fevers crushed my head like a steamroller. So, on the rare occasions when Joey wasn't there and the narcotics wore off, I simply couldn't wait for the call bell to be answered and hauled myself, I.V. cart in tow, down the hall to the nurse's station to plead for immediate drugs like a pathetic heroine addict.

To make things worse, a yellow radioactive sign hung like an insult, on the outside of my room door to warn passersby of what was inside - me on chemotherapy. On occasion I'd forget that the sign was there, but when the door flung open, I'd see it. In the haze of my feverish brain I'd think that I too needed to get away from the area. One time I fantasized that I'd tie the sheets together to escape from the window like an episode of I Love Lucy.

Joey camped out by my bedside, slept in an uncomfortable chair, and worked from his laptop and cell phone. He left only for trips to

Starbucks for me, much tastier food for the both of us, home for clean clothes for him and my monument papers so that I could write some more. In general, I felt like a freak, grieved for the abuse heaped upon my poor body, and hoped that whatever the problem was, it'd be cleared up before graduate school in August.

In my pursuit to strike a better balance, I knew what made me happy and the pursuit of higher education was at the top of my list. I've had a life-long passion for literature and one of my goals is to teach at the college level. Throughout the years, incredible professors have inspired me and encouraged me to write. Before The Cancer Monument, I hardly knew what to do with myself for the few weeks in between school semesters and couldn't wait for the next semester to begin. I love the smell and feel of walls of books at the library. I crave intellectual conversations about the history of ideas and the influence of great American writers and poets like Hawthorne, Poe, Twain, Faulkner, Frost, Morrison, and Angelou. A Masters degree was a long-ago requirement that I'd set for myself and despite my illness, I wasn't about to sacrifice it because of cancer. More than anything, I just wanted to be healthy again. Finally, on the third day, a leading infectious disease specialist, back from a trip to Africa, came to tell Joey and me the reason why I was in the hospital.

"What the hell is wrong with me?" I asked the doctor.

"It's a Staph infection," the doctor said. "You're very lucky that the hospital continued to pump you with antibiotics otherwise you'd be dead right now."

I didn't know anything about Staph then, but once the doctor explained, I felt like I'd walked away from the guillotine. A Staph infection got into my medi-port and it frightened me to learn just how common that was. Staph was deadly and people died within a day if untreated. I still felt like a wildcat with a burr on my tail about the eleven E.R. needle sticks in the chest, but I was grateful to be alive.

I had lots of visitors while I was in the hospital, including my oncologist, Dr. Smith, who came to tell me that two rounds of chemotherapy shrunk my tumor by fifty percent. We were making good progress against cancer, but still had four more months of chemo to go. My Department Director at work also stopped by to visit and assured me that despite the corporate merger in progress, my job was safe, my application for a promotion was still in the running and most importantly, I was valued and needed at work. I hadn't cried about too much since my diagnosis a couple of months earlier, but at this news, I couldn't hold back tears. I now felt safer in the world and expressed how grateful I was for her visit. I worked for a major wireless telecommunications company and though it wasn't my dream to work there until retirement, the relief and knowledge of a job with benefits was a priceless treasure to me. Joey and I were excited with all the good news and after a week in the hospital and three more weeks of daily intravenous antibiotics, so strong that it could've clean city streets, the Staph was gone, but of course, cancer remained. Joey and I were excited for brighter days ahead and hoped that 2001 would be a much better year.

***

Since the beginning of chemotherapy, my menstrual cycles stopped and a chemo-induced menopause, complete with head-to-toe hot flashes began. The fact that I was in a state of menopause never occurred to me and wasn't diagnosed until months later. For the first time since sixth grade, I actually wished for that timely visitor to return just so that I'd have a measure of normalcy back in my life. One minute, I'd cry hysterically about a tiny spider on its way across the living room floor and the next, I'd practically tear Joey's head off like a she-devil wielding bizarre hormonal lunacy against steady logic. Hot flashes woke me up at all hours of the night to soaked pajamas and during the day my mascara lost its waterproof claim and streaked down my face as I presided over meetings at work. I'd fantasize about cleaving off my volcanic breasts just to find relief from the tender pain and could often be found seated in front of an open freezer wishing it were possible to lay next to the frozen green beans and chopped meat. Bald, bloated from medicines, and hormonally imbalanced in the heat of a triple-digit Texas summer, I continued to struggle with self-image issues and by my thirty-fourth birthday that summer, I felt ugly, old, and undesirable.

Once I shared this information with my doctor, I was only slightly comforted by the fact that the lack of a cycle was considered normal for many women on chemo, and that this chemo-induced menopause would likely be a temporary condition. So, with the promise of a future in sight, Joey and I talked about starting our own family once I was in remission and my menstrual cycles returned. After the Staph infection was over, we scheduled a visit to see a fertility specialist to obtain further information and establish a post-cancer plan of action. In all of the craziness of the first couple of months of cancer: the life and death issues, the possibility of organ failure, the security of my job, health insurance, and our wedding plans, fertility didn't make the cut of immediate concerns to be addressed.

"Chemotherapy attacks the rapidly growing cells, like hair and cancer cells," the fertility doctor explained to us. We'd been told this before and were relieved to hear consistency. We were also glad to learn that ovaries weren't among the rapidly growing cells. Again, the fertility specialist repeated the words of my oncologist when he said that I'd entered "a temporary chemo-induced menopause." Nature would return once I had time to heal as it had for so many women who had babies after cancer, but he cautioned, there were no guarantees.

So, once I finished with treatments, the plan was to monitor my hormone levels and hopefully normalcy would return. That was the plan anyway. But, just in case my cycle didn't return, Joey and I discussed plans B, C and D. There were lots of options for infertile couples, but once we dug deeper to unravel their ambiguities, many were ones that we'd never consider. Still, we felt overwhelmed with all the choices and considered it to be a moot point if I couldn't have my health back, or worse, was dead. We thought it best to put the entire topic of parenthood on the back burner until the time was right and looked forward to a future that would include children, but considered our lives with no children, too. Whatever the final outcome, it'd be a choice that we would make together and one that would create balance and harmony in our lives. It was in God's hands anyway so we decided to live with joy and purpose in the meantime.

Laura Freer, my manager at work had become my friend along the way. Like many women, Laura continuously strove to strike a balance between her career, motherhood to three boys under the age of five, which included a set of twins, marriage, and somehow, time for herself. Before my cancer diagnosis, Laura and I talked many times about the daily struggles, anxieties, and expectations of being a woman and how the need for balance was difficult to achieve when we were pulled in so many directions.

The life-long socialization process of women began from birth and forced a myriad of behaviors and beliefs, including the beauty quotient. As a former fashion model, Laura knew firsthand the detriments of the beauty factor which teaches females that worth and success are determined by the ability to achieve a front-cover standard of beauty. Laura and I discussed these many issues as well as the fine line between being successful and just being a bitch. Boundaries with others can be difficult to establish because as women, we have to be many things to many people and sometimes boundaries are blurred: a loyal friend, daughter, sister, wife, mother, co-worker, a good neighbor, and in most all of these situations we're required to smile through unfairness, be helpful, understand, forgive at all times, be nice to everyone, and no matter what, look great too. Now in our thirties, Laura and I knew the game a lot better than we did in our twenties and we were tired of it all. Now that I had cancer, these previous conversations with Laura were more pertinent to me than ever. It was time for me to establish better boundaries and balance. You have to do this, or else be devoured whole by the situation, I thought one day as I sat at my desk. Beginning was the hardest part.

My co-workers became my first test subjects in my efforts to establish better balance. Cancer is a strange entity and even has the ability to influence polite people to abandon their basic manners. To others it seemed that a red neon sign flashed over my head as if to announce: I have cancer, please say anything to me. My co-workers asked intrusive questions and I was expected to answer them all with exuberance. I didn't want to share details of my personal life with my co-workers and there was no law that required me to do so. I wanted to come to work and do the job that I was hired to do, but now because of my cancer, the social aspects of the work environment were at times without boundaries.

Eventually, I'd find my way through the maze, but until such time, I experienced many incidences of rudeness, ignorance, and outright cruelty. Not only would people feel free to infringe upon my private life with a mask of sincerity and blatantly sensationalize my crisis for their own bizarre pleasure, but no matter what personal accomplishments I'd share with them beyond the scope of cancer, some still insisted on viewing me on their terms; to them above all else, I was a pitiful cancer victim.

When I was first diagnosed, Laura and I decided that a meeting with those that I worked the closest with was a good idea. I was unprepared for the fact that they were more upset about my cancer than I was. In general, they were frightened for me and felt helpless to know how to help me. With a business-as-usual attitude, I answered their questions, explained as much as I knew, told them what to expect, and reassured them that I planned to beat cancer. They were comforted with all of this information, but every now and then when we talked, they'd burst out in tears.

"Why are you crying?" I'd ask in a state of confused frustration. It'd be one thing if I was actually crying in front of them, but I wasn't.

"It's just so sad," they'd say, "I can't believe you have cancer when you look so normal." It was bizarre that I had to console them when

I wasn't upset, but I was learning that people's emotions are highly unpredictable in crisis.

"Well, I'm just as shocked as you are by everything but there's a plan in place, I'm on track, and I'll be fine. If anything, this stresses the importance of early diagnosis." I said. I'd found my classroom of students to teach. It wasn't the great works of Shakespeare or Hemingway, but over time I heard the stories of how my cancer caused a ripple effect of awareness with my co-workers. Many were inspired to get physicals, or made their spouses get a physical. One person had a strange mole examined, a few got first-time mammograms, and one co-worker stopped smoking. Though I was on chemo, I'd remain quite independent throughout, though at a much slower pace than before.

Sensing that my co-workers needed to feel needed, I promised that I wouldn't hesitate to ask for help though I emphasized that I was the same person with many interests beyond the scope of cancer. I let them know too that cancer was not the death sentence that it once was and that many people were now cancer-free because of modern medicine and lived healthy, normal lives for decades after their bout with cancer. Tears were not my method of resolution and I told my co-workers that if only for my benefit, they should do likewise when around me.

I didn't mind sharing personal information with this close-knit group because their sincerity was evident. They truly wanted to help me and wanted to understand more about the subject of cancer, which they knew nothing about except only for fear and death. I was their first up-close and personal experience with this ugly plague and was glad to be a resource of information for them while we all took a journey through Cancer Land. After a while, they saw the routine and even when a few bumps and stones were thrown in the road, I was generally calm and methodical, which made them better able to cope with cancer too. We soon got back to a regular work routine with fewer long-winded conversations about cancer and they remained my continuous emotional support team.

The rest of the office audience was not so easy to figure out, especially a small band of ignorant fools that we called "the vultures." For them, my marriage, sex life, cancer treatments, and future became a water cooler cliffhanger. I was under no obligation to share personal information or talk about my illness with anyone, ever, but was willing to do so for the sake of prevention. It wasn't clear to me that the vultures wanted to be educated and without a motivated student, a teacher's job is made more difficult. I'm not sure what this group expected to see as they stretched their necks to catch a glimpse of the cancer victim.

However, it was evident that I'd gone from a private, hard-working person to one that could scarcely get more than ten minutes of work in at a time. One, or all in this flock of fowl would stop by my desk under the guise of a good-natured chat. At times, I felt like sideshow at a carnival, vulnerable to the indiscriminate ignorance of an unsophisticated, low priced audience who craved oddity and gore. The fifty questions a day coupled with the hardships and threats of cancer added to my stress and lack of normalcy. To adapt to various situations, I learned to project different personas to handle these unsolicited bands of curiosity-seekers and questionable do-gooders. There was the policeman at the highway accident whose attitude was something like this: "Move it along people, there's nothing to see here." Or, in certain situations the publicist persona might be required: "Michelle is currently unavailable. Due to an overwhelming response, we will not be able to acknowledge every inquiry. Thank you for your support!" My favorite persona was the efficiency expert where the economy of time and a streamlined process meant everything. I learned the power of the delete key when people sent me unwelcome emails. I screened my calls more than ever and let voice mail work for me. If you made an in-person visit and your agenda wasn't clear in the first one minute, I'd help you to it and if akin to a death fugue, or other unnecessary negative scenario, I stood up, thanked you, and ushered you, or myself away from the scene. It's not that I refused to talk about cancer at work, I did so with great regularity, but it was the gravitation towards the morose and unproductive that I preferred to avoid so that I could stay focused, limit my stress, maintain my dignity, and find a balance within my crisis.

This new pattern took weeks to establish, but eventually people learned my expectations of them and also realized that I was the same person, only with cancer. People learned not to come around unless their reasons were clear, productive, and not at my expense. Others soon stayed away completely, which was fine by me, and actually, I felt quite accomplished in my new boundary-making policies. Eventually, I came to realize that it wasn't me they verbally attacked; it was cancer itself. Bound in fear and without adequate answers from science, it was easier for some to blame the victim than to accept the frightening reality that there was no cure, or perhaps they might be the next person in line for chemotherapy.

Crisis brings out our true characters. Action is required in crisis. What we meant to do, or wanted to say is irrelevant because in the final analysis, words and deeds are the measure of a human being. In the face of urgent circumstances, our motivations and intentions can no longer be masked. The false-hearted are flushed out of their dark holes of indifference, and denial is no longer possible. In crisis, our ethics are tested, forced into action, and opportunities to show mercy and compassion exist. Crisis is where the teachings of our youth, the experiences of our pasts converge, faith is tested, and our integrity is on the line for all to see.

From the view of my desk at work and in hospital waiting rooms, I'd continue to see varied responses to cancer and with it, saw the human extremes of generosity and brutal ignorance among society at large. That year, I came to know the story of a woman named Denise in South Carolina whose boss, a man named Bob, battled cancer. Denise shared with me her innermost discoveries about coping with cancer, the nature of people, and life in general, all of which she learned as a result of Bob's journey.

Denise didn't always get along with Bob. He was her office manager who had a smart aleck quip for everything, which made it difficult for anyone to know him on a personal level. Two weeks before his daughter's wedding, Bob complained about his neck hurting, but everyone shrugged it off to the type of fatherly stress associated with pre-wedding circumstances. Six years earlier, Bob had been cured of Malignant Melanoma with an experimental procedure. But now, as the pain in his neck mounted to an intolerable level, he had an MRI; later that day the results revealed the worst.

While at her desk, Denise heard a man's tearful voice and knew that Bob's MRI results were not good. His specific words were inaudible, but she felt his pain from across the room and her instincts told her to run to him and tell him it would be all right. Instead, Denise sat frozen at her desk and did not know how to help.

"Our boss, our leader was crying and it all seemed so overwhelming to me," she said. "I discussed the matter with another co-worker. We both felt helpless. We all seemed to scatter, unwilling and too frightened to face the truth that Bob had cancer."

Moments later, Bob composed himself and told his staff that Melanoma had come back with a vengeance and was in his lung and brain. Denise took notice of her co-workers in the room. Each one extended a hand, or offered a prayer to comfort him, but it was a mechanical gesture made without real emotion. Denise could no longer contain her emotion and threw her arms around Bob. She held him like a brother and they cried together. The other co-workers had already returned to their desks. By 5:00 p.m., Bob went home and Denise did too and found no peace.

Denise couldn't believe cancer was happening again to Bob, who was such a vibrant and talented person. In a weird way, she felt that she'd received the diagnosis herself, though she hadn't.

"How was I going to cope with this horrible tragedy every day? How could I be strong for myself, and Bob? I have only surface knowledge of the different types of cancer such as Melanoma," she thought. Denise soon realized that in order to function in her new crisis, she needed more information and began to research for hours on the Internet about Melanoma. She shared her findings with Bob about the latest treatments to encourage him not to give up hope for a cure. Weeks later, Bob met with his co-workers again to reassure them that he intended to beat his disease. With brave tears in his eyes, he told them that he intended to fight cancer with all that he had, but said that, "...if he lost the battle, he would win the war on the other side with our Lord." His co-workers sat in stony silence and barely made eye contact with one another.

Bob's work defined him and gave him great satisfaction. He wanted to continue working as long as he could, but knowing that he was about to begin radiation to his brain, he distributed out his job duties among the staff, uncertain of his outcome. To Denise and others, it signaled another step in the reality that Bob's life was coming to an end. Every day at the office, Denise's heart was filled with pain as she watched a powerful man be reduced by the ravenous strongholds of cancer. Absolutely no one deserved to die this unfairly, she thought. Added to this grief was the stunning lack of compassion and superficiality of the other co-workers towards Bob, and this angered Denise. She began to notice that certain co-workers avoided the path to Bob's office and then Bob all together, saying that they: "couldn't bring themselves to speak to him for fear of crying in front of him."

Denise tried to reason that their fear was really about a selfish awareness of their own mortality that kept them from giving much needed comfort to a dying man. Strangely, Denise's co-workers still wanted to know the details of the situation without really being involved, and knowing that Bob and Denise had forged a new chapter in their relationship since his illness, they'd frequently sidle up to her for the latest details.

"I thought my co-workers were a bunch of cowards by this time," Denise told me, but she still had to go to work with them so she kept her responses factual, but brief, and her anger unspoken.

Soon, the man that Denise once knew as Bob began to change inside and out. Bob's sassy, sometimes arrogant attitude fled like a thief in the night, and a gentle, kind and humble man was born. Steroid medication helped to ease the pain in his neck and caused him to look bloated. His hair began to slowly fall out from radiation and as he walked down the hall one afternoon, Denise recalled that a clump seemed to sadly slip away like a snowman in the sun. Bob was proud of his appearance and though he was terminally ill, he still wanted to look and feel good about himself so he began to wear a stylish hat.

Unlike her co-workers who seemed to still hold a grudge for Bob's past slights, Denise couldn't ignore the fact that Bob was a human being in great need of care and compassion as he faced death. Soon Denise became depressed about her co-workers' lack of compassion, but refused to remain powerless and sought other ways to help Bob and his family without being intrusive. With her Internet research she read that blueberries carried cancer-fighting antioxidants and that chocolate did, too. When blueberries finally appeared on the five bushes in her back yard, she stood among the mosquitoes and picked them bare so that she could bring them to Bob. She brought Bob his favorite Snickers Bar every week and sent him a thoughtful card to inspire him and let him know that he was wanted and needed in the world. Both Bob and his wife enjoyed these cards and Denise enjoyed sending them too. Denise no longer felt helpless about cancer because she knew that her actions made a difference in Bob's life and maybe, just maybe, she hoped to love him back to health again.

Bob needed friendship. He needed to talk about so many things and together he and Denise discussed what he held dear to him in life: his wife, children, and church. He talked about people in general, how he wished that he'd known those around him better before he became ill, and how he wished for more time to make a difference. Bob's eyes filled with tears as he said that he wanted everyone to know what good had come from his illness. He had a renewed sense of spirit and now knew what was truly important in life.

"I didn't get it before; I do now," he said to Denise one day. "It isn't what you wear or who you are in life. What's important is church and family."

Bob's children were a great source of pride to him and as he viewed his daughter's wedding video one day with his wife he said, "I complained about the cost of the wedding, but look at her smile. Look at her happiness. The memory of that day far outweighs any cost."

As Bob's body grew weaker from cancer and cancer treatments his days at the office grew fewer too. He was a proud man and wanted no help getting up the stairs, but when he was no longer able to drive, he accepted help from two co-workers who gladly picked him up and took him home every day. Through it all, he kept his sense of humor intact and wanted everyone to treat him as they had before. He was still Bob, the guy that loved to laugh, joke, and tell stories.

By this time all the employees were more guarded around Bob and avoided negative topics. Denise noticed a kinder side to her co-workers as they showed great humanity towards Bob, who was dying rapidly. Still, a few co-workers remained reserved, unable to forgive past disagreements with Bob, and retreated to the isolation of their icy hearts. Denise felt sorry for them, not Bob. Fully and completely, Bob gave the last bits of himself: his wit, his intelligence, and even his smart-aleck quips. Denise, too, had previous work disagreements with Bob, but all that was in the past now.

Five months had passed since Bob's cancer diagnosis and despite his doctor's advice and the urging of everyone else for him to enjoy his time and leave work altogether, he stayed and held his post. He'd taken only one weekend in the previous months to go to the mountains and watch the eagles soar. Finally, Bob's last day at work arrived and as Denise walked into his office, it seemed impossible to her that he'd never sit at his desk again.

The next time she saw Bob it was a few days later at his hospital bedside as his entire family held a vigil around him. Despite his fight for air and deteriorated condition, he found it necessary to maintain dignity and manners enough to introduce Denise to everyone. Bob's life had come down to final moments and his personal war against cancer was about to be won. Denise kissed his forehead for the first and last time. Then, in that sudden moment, Denise said that she knew beyond any doubt, she saw Bob's soul and he saw hers too.

Because of Bob's death, Denise saw life differently than ever before. The day after his passing, some co-workers suggested that a Remembrance Book be made in honor of Bob and to be given to his family. Only a few seemed interested to participate or share the expenses, so Denise decided to take responsibility for the project. She asked that her co-workers write a note, poem, or memory of Bob and was dumbfounded to meet opposition from a few. To make the Remembrance Book, Denise traveled to places that Bob loved. She took pictures and collected seashells and after putting the book together she came to the following conclusions, which helped her grieve and cope:

"Cancer in any form is a horrible disease however within the journey of cancer can be found limitless opportunities for both the diagnosed and the healthy to access the power of their human spirits on this side of the living. The experience of facing death opens our eyes and hearts and allows for kindness where bitterness once roamed and offers us all the opportunity for hope, renewal and a sense of purpose."

The very last picture in Bob's Remembrance Book was a bald eagle, a great American symbol of strength and power. Denise smiled to think that Bob, too, was now like the eagle, a free spirit who soared to a place greater than us all.

***

Hope. It had become a strange word to me and from the moment of my cancer diagnosis it was thrown around as if everyone knew exactly what it meant. But for me, and the many others that I'd meet along the way, hope in the face of cancer proved to be as malleable as molten lava and as unpredictable as the path of a tornado.

One day, some of my co-workers and I went to lunch at a favorite all-u-can eat sushi buffet. Though my doctor would've had a fit to know that I ate raw fish with low white-blood counts, that day it was my prescription for fun. I hoped to make it through lunch without hearing a reference made to cancer, whether directly or indirectly, but it was impossible. Somewhere between the squid salad, spicy raw scallops, and sea urchin the conversation gravitated to the inevitable topic: cancer.

Her mouth full of seaweed, one of my co-workers motioned with chopsticks to sputter out well-intentioned advice, "God never gives you more than you can handle. You just have to believe that you'll get better. Attitude is everything."

It was a statement of hope and on most days I really believed it too. But that day, I thought remarks like that were a giant load of fairy tale crap. That day, it didn't feel like God cared about me at all. For the sake of my co-workers, I held my tongue because I realized that they needed to believe that I believed. So, I sat through the rest of lunch and made polite conversation as idealistic concepts like hope, faith, positive attitude and others jumbled in my mind and gave me a whopper headache. I thought I'd always known the meaning of these important words and now it all seemed like bull. I wondered if God would hurl a tidal wave at me next just to see if I could handle it.

Over time, I'd meet many people on the front line of the War on Cancer and their levels of hope for a cure were phenomenal and their faith in God was so steady that cancer seemed no match. Despite it all, for some, cancer had the upper hand and in the end, their only hope left was the right to claim a beautiful death. Yes, hope was a tricky word for me then, but later I'd come to know the incredible stories of Heroes like Justin and Charles whose incredible love and bravery inspired me.

At work, a woman named Ginger was among the new employees hired as a result of the corporate merger. It didn't take long for word to get to her that I had cancer. She took an immediate caregiver role that at first stunned me. Her voice was soothing and maternal and it was easy to let go long enough to accept help from her. Behind Ginger's smile, she wore a concerned gaze and a face heavy with sadness. I figured she was worried that I'd die so I tried to reassure her that I'd be okay. Ginger didn't say how or why, but she seemed to know exactly what I was going through. She doted on me in a variety of little ways that made being at work more comfortable. She brought me herbal teas, granola bars and when I couldn't find a spoon for my yogurt one day, she scoured high and low to find one, and then made sure that a box of plastic utensils were in her desk drawer for me at all times. Everything about Ginger was sincere and loving. We became trusted friends and a year later she told me about Justin.

A mother's heart is sometimes a tormented place, mixed with unconditional love, nightmarish fears, unfailing hope, and silent prayers to anyone in heaven who will listen. When Ginger's first child was born she named him Justin, and was filled with immense happiness. As she held her baby boy close to smell the newness of his skin and to trace the perfect shape of his mouth, the joys of first time motherhood were unlike any feelings she'd ever experienced. Justin was a perfect child in every way and as a new mother Ginger finally understood her purpose in the world.

"I felt that surely, this had to be paradise," she told me. In Justin's first few months of life their bonds were forged as Ginger sang her son to sleep with made up lullaby songs that reflected the flood of joy in her heart. As Justin lay quietly sleeping next to her she'd whisper in his ear all the many wonderful things she planned to show and teach him.

Never did Ginger imagine that nine years later, an inoperable brain stem Glioma would take Justin's life. More than fifteen years have passed since Justin died. Coping with the loss is still difficult for Ginger, but sharing her story helps to keep her son's memory alive, and eases the pain of grief just a little.

"My hope is that by sharing my story, others may have a raised awareness about cancer and how to cope with loss in the best way possible," Ginger says. "There is never an easy way to make sense of a child's death, but there is much to learn from these heroic, courageous, insightful little ones who sit dangling on the fence of life, or death. My remaining months with Justin as mother and son consisted of lessons in dying as I taught him, not about how to safely cross the street, but how to cross over into the Light on the way to his new life in heaven."

Justin was an ordinary kid who loved planes and dreamed of being a Navy pilot when he grew up. Ginger was surprised when his teacher phoned one day to say that he'd been having difficulty seeing the blackboard. She sought professional advice, but the reasons were unknown and rapidly worsened. Justin was soon wearing an eye patch over one eye, and from that point forward, things quickly sped out of control. Tests soon revealed that the cause for his vision problem was a brain tumor and a sentence of terminal cancer was handed out. The doctors could do nothing to save Justin, though they tried with a combination of radiation and steroids.

"Our family tried to save Justin too. With every atom in our collective beings we tried to love him back into health and made many, many desperate prayers to God," Ginger told me.

Every day, Ginger took Justin to the hospital for cancer treatments. She also had two daughters; an infant and one in elementary school. Ginger said that every moment of that time in her life was like living on the edge of cliff, but somehow she found the strength to shift into automatic pilot for the sake of her children. Life was often a mechanical existence filled with a myriad of daily phone calls, meals, diaper changes, laundry, and the countless daily duties of being a wife and mother. She wanted to spend every moment with Justin so that his mind would be flooded with beautiful memories to last them until they'd meet again in heaven.

In the newness of the crisis, close relatives, and kind neighbors helped in the best way they could. The greatest form of help, Ginger could not have - to make her son whole and healthy again.

"Justin's death sentence had been handed out and was spread upon our plates to eat slowly each day as our family helplessly watched him deteriorate and die," Ginger said.

She punished herself with the inevitable questions: What did I do wrong? Am I being punished for some guilty offense committed in my youth? Ginger's daughters were healthy and so was the rest of the family. So, why was Justin the only person with cancer? No one would ever know. Cancer treatments did very little to help minimize the brain tumor and were also increasingly difficult on Justin's little body.

He was not unaware of the drastic changes in his appearance due to steroids and one evening while looking at a photo of himself taken in healthier days he asked his mother, "Mommy, will I ever look like this again?"

"Yes," Ginger told him, but she knew that it would be in heaven.

As Justin's cancer progressed, Ginger knew that she'd have to talk to her son about death. Finally, the subject couldn't be avoided and as Justin sat in his wheelchair, breathing with the help of an oxygen tank, and almost completely blind from the growing pressure of the tumor, Ginger talked to Justin about heaven.

"Justin," she asked, "do you think that maybe you won't get well?"

"No," he said, "I'll get well."

"Sometimes, Mommy thinks that maybe you might not get better and that this cancer might make you die." Looking up at his mother Justin said,

"No, I know that God won't let me die." He reached up to hug his mother with both arms and said, "It will be okay, no matter what happens." Ginger was humbled to realize that Justin was consoling her.

"He didn't want me to be sad," Ginger told me in amazement. "He understood his fate, and he felt a responsibility to make me at peace with his destiny like he was."

Very soon after, Justin lost his speech, but he was still very aware of his surroundings and Ginger offered him the earthly things he loved best to help him hold on to life just a little while longer. Ginger remembers that Justin never complained once about the pain or even about the fact that he was dying. During this time too there were lots of visitors: family, friends, neighbors and curiosity seekers descended, most with sincere intentions, but a small few soon revealed hidden personal agendas like one person, who took notes for her Masters degree in Psychology. She was promptly escorted off the premises.

Then one day, a neighbor's rudeness blind-sided Ginger as the conversation shifted to an unbelievable question, "...she asked me if I would have another child after Justin died as though he could be replaced like a lost puppy," Ginger recalled in disbelief.

Ginger also began to notice that other visitors had a peculiar, exploitive interest to see a dying little boy as though he were a highway accident to slow down, gawk, and gossip about on front porches and around dinner tables. Blunt comments led to pointed blame and before she knew it, once sympathetic people told Ginger outright that she'd somehow caused her son's illness or even more strangely, that she was paying for some wrong she'd committed in a past life. These hurtful comments did little to help Ginger cope with the approaching death of her son. Those people in her life who were on the more positive side of religion offered clichéd answers for why God takes little children back to heaven. Ginger didn't want to hear any of it. Time was running out. Her boy was dying and it couldn't be explained or ignored so she pushed all of the chatter aside and focused on the job at hand, being Justin's mother and vowed that until his last breath, she'd love and protect him.

Ginger was afraid that Justin might hear the negative comments from others and put an end to all visitors, except for the immediate family. Only love was allowed to enter into the sanctity of their space. Justin was now so weak and every movement, even a simple conversation, or smile took every bit of energy he possessed. Those who had seemed to care so much before no longer called Ginger, sent a card, dropped off a tuna casserole, or offered her a ride to the hospital, but the family continued to live in their crisis and coped as best as possible.

After Justin lost his speech, he grew steadily weaker. Soon he couldn't swallow and had to be suctioned just to help him breathe. Finally, Ginger agreed to have the nurses administer morphine and in that moment, she explained to me how incredibly conflicted she felt. She didn't want her son to die, nor did she want him suffer to his death, but the idea that she was somehow assisting his death was a very difficult concept when she was his mother and had given him life. But for Justin's sake, Ginger could not dwell on this thought. She loved her son and the only hope that remained was to give him a peaceful death, to sleep, and feel no pain as he died.

Then, on September 5th, the day of Justin's death, his breathing was rhythmic and Ginger knew that it was just a matter of time before God would take him from her. She called all who loved Justin to his bedside to say goodbye. Ginger believes that though Justin couldn't communicate, he heard them all. She never left Justin's side. As his breathing grew shallow she became aware of time unlike never before. She wanted to grab the air, somehow, capture the seconds and fling them all backwards for more moments with her son. Ginger knew that she couldn't keep Justin any longer when heaven wanted him too.

Ginger told her son that it was his time to go. "I told him that we'd miss him, but we'd be all right. I promised to take good care of his sisters and gave him his final instructions to follow the Light to the other side as he made his way to heaven. Then, I bent over his beautiful, peaceful face and softly said, 'It's time, Justin. Go fly your plane.' With those words, he took his last breath and quietly died."

For several years after Justin's death military jets flew directly over his house. Ginger told her daughters that it was Justin, just passing by to say hello.

"We'd look up to the sky and say, 'Go fly your plane Justin'," Ginger smiled.

Helping her daughters cope with Justin's death has been a challenge for Ginger through the years, especially during the holidays. Though they can't see or touch Justin, they never forget him and never avoid the topic of his death if it is mentioned. Many times, Ginger goes to the attic when no one is home to go through Justin's things, the only physical reminders that he was once a little boy. Up there alone, Ginger reads through the cards and letters that people sent during his illness and even some from strangers who read about him in the newspaper.

To this day, Ginger is left with so many unanswered questions: Are we all living life by chance? Or, is there a master plan and grander purpose for each of us to teach and be taught by the human joys and sufferings of one another on this earth? The answers wouldn't become clearer with the passage of time, but the pain in her heart is eased a little with the notion that her son's life and death can somehow help and heal others.

One year after Justin's death, his friend Chris also died of cancer. Chris' parents had tremendous difficulty releasing their son to heaven and he hung on to life because of it. Ginger was with Chris during his last moments of breath when he spoke about Justin being in the room. Ginger believes that her little boy was in the room that day to help his friend, as his mommy had once helped him, cross over to the Light on the way to heaven.

***

No matter how aggressive cancer can be it can never destroy the timeless bonds of love. On numerous occasions, I was reminded of this lesson from the cancer heroes around me, including a man named Charles. Charles battled in both the Korean and Vietnam Wars, and for 50 years Luci was his one and only sweetheart. Charles wasn't the type to fear his tender side. He embraced it. To his wife and children, he was a great leader and protector who often referred to the Bible verse from I Corinthians 13:1-13 as both a life lesson and a reminder that in the end, nothing else mattered except for love. Through the years, he not only spoke these words of love, but also showed his family in numerous ways how much he loved them. Between him and Luci, one such way became known as the "special spot." Long ago, Charles designated a special, secret area in the house that only he and Luci knew about. In this place, he'd leave her a little love token: a note, or a piece of candy and one time he left a ring from a gumball machine just for fun.

"Have you looked in your special spot?" he'd ask. Then, Luci would check her special spot to discover what had been left for her. But in the bustle of life, Luci sometimes forgot to check her special spot for long stretches at a time, to which Charles would inquire, "Have you looked in your special spot lately?"

"Oh!" Luci would exclaim, "Not in a long while!" Later on that day, after the dinner was cooked, dishes put away and the children put to bed, she'd go to her special spot to see what Charles had left for her and with each thoughtful token she rediscovered why he was her beloved.

One day, everything changed. Charles began to experience swollen ankles to the point that he sought medical attention. Since he was seventy-two years old, the doctor attributed it to old age and prescribed a diuretic to release the water retention. Next, came persistent nausea, which sent the family to the emergency room where Luci insisted that Charles have a CT scan. However, the doctor didn't call them with the results and Charles' condition worsened.

Finally, the family demanded answers and on his daughter's birthday, Charles and his family sat squeezed in the tiny examination room to learn the results of the CT scan. The doctor entered and held their fate on a piece of paper. Then, the unforgettable words: terminal cancer. Charles had pancreatic cancer, with a metastasis to his liver and was told that he had between two weeks to two months to live. Everyone was stunned.

In the car ride home, silence hung as each person retreated to deep thoughts. It didn't make sense. It wasn't fair. In only a few months, he and Luci would celebrate their 50th wedding anniversary. He still hadn't experienced being a great-grandpa. Life couldn't be over when there was still more to experience. Without warning, consultation, or permission, his lifetime had now been redefined and time was now measured in weeks, days, hours, minutes, and moments.

After surviving battle in two wars, Charles would now fight in one more, this time against an unseen cancer enemy, which had silently gained much ground against him. Within days, he was on chemotherapy in the hope that his life might be prolonged enough to find a research drug and a cure. The entire family experienced a range of emotions from fear, anger to disbelief and finally, acceptance. They held to their faith and prayed daily for a miracle.

"In the end nothing else matters except for love," he reminded his daughter, Carolyn, one day as they drove home from the cancer center. Each moment was more precious than ever now and was filled with love, laughter and memories as they held out hope but also planned for a funeral. Just as Charles was involved in the process of his life, so too was he involved in the process of his death and asked his daughter to read the Corinthians passage as his eulogy and testament to his life. Two weeks and two months passed, then three months.

Charles slipped into a coma during the first days of November. His eyes clouded over. He was silent. His family sensed that the end was near. On November 7th, their golden wedding anniversary, Luci went to her husband's bedside,

"Happy anniversary…you made it. I love you," she said.

Suddenly, Charles opened his eyes, which were now clear and bright. "I love you," he said. He closed his eyes, slipped back into a coma, and died a week later.

As if tears from heaven, the rain poured on the day of Charles' funeral. As instructed, Carolyn read her father's eulogy:

> "If I speak in the tongues of mortals and of angels, but do not have love, I am a noisy gong or a clanging cymbal. And if I have prophetic powers, and understand all mysteries and all knowledge, and if I have all faith, so as to remove mountains, but do not have love, I am nothing. If I give away all my possessions, and if I hand over my body so that I may boast, but do not have love, I gain nothing. Love is patient; love is kind; love is not envious or boastful or arrogant or rude. It does not insist on its own way; it is not irritable or resentful; it does not rejoice in wrongdoing, but rejoices in the truth. It bears all things, believes all things, hopes all things, endures all things. Love never ends. But as for prophecies, they will come to an end; as for tongues, they will cease; as for knowledge, it will come to an end.

For we know only in part, and we prophesy only in part; but when the complete comes, the partial will come to an end. When I was a child, I spoke like a child, I thought like a child, I reasoned like a child; when I became an adult, I put an end to childish ways. For now we see in a mirror, dimly, but then we will see face to face. Now I know only in part; then I will know fully, even as I have been fully known. And now faith, hope, and love abide, these three; and the greatest of these is love."

(I Corinthians 13: 1-13)

The process of grief is unpredictable and slow. Months after Charles' death, Luci went to sleep one night and in a dream her husband came to ask, "Have you looked in your special spot lately?" Charles held out his hand to show his beloved a diamond anniversary ring. Luci awoke, stunned that her husband had spoken to her in a dream. For months after Charles' death, she dreamt of him several times, but never did he speak. Now, his presence was so real, his words so strong that she couldn't shrug it off to the process of grief.

Could there really be something in her special spot, she wondered. It had been so long since the last time she'd checked it. Surely, it had to be empty, she thought. A part of her felt kind of silly, after all, it was just a dream, she told herself. Luci's heart pounded with a mixture of curious hope and as she slowly looked inside her special spot her eyes could not believe that something was inside! Wrapped inside a note was the exact ring that Charles showed her in the dream. The note? It said: I love you.

This incredible surprise filled the family with great amazement and joy. They laughed to imagine what Charles, now in heaven, must have thought about the undiscovered ring: "Is she ever going to find that diamond ring? For Pete's sake, looks like I'll have to tell her about it or else it'll stay there forever!"

In all of the commotion of a cancer diagnosis, the physical crush of chemo and the last minute preparations of trying to end a life with dignity, purpose and care, Charles managed to purchase the diamond anniversary ring without anyone knowing about it. Over the years, the special spot provided a lifetime of love tokens and cherished memories between the giver and receiver alike. Now, not even the boundaries of death could prevent another; a diamond ring and a timeless message from heaven to last forever.

Some months later in February, the family attended Sunday church services. It was also Charles' birthday, and in the month best known for love, the priest fashioned his sermon from an appropriate source, which filled them all with awe - I Corinthians 13:1-13.

***

How do I get through cancer? I had asked myself that question from the very beginning and still, no one handed me a compass. Yet, coping remained a daily requirement for me as necessary as food and water. As I'd continue to search for new strategies to get to the next point in my journey, more cancer stories filled me with inspiration including the stories of Amy, Celeste, and Arvid.

Amy was diagnosed with breast cancer one week after her 35th birthday. By chance she happened to feel a tiny lump on her right breast when she applied sunscreen one day. Two doctors considered the lump benign because it wasn't hard and solid, 'the usual consistency of a regular tumor,' they said.

"Wait three months," one doctor said. "Then we'll be able to tell if the tumor has changed in size."

Amy didn't want to wait. "What would you do if I were your wife?" she questioned back. She didn't know what came over her; she wasn't the type to be so bold, especially to a doctor, but, she was a mother of two children and they counted on her to stay alive. So within days, a biopsy was done and a breast cancer diagnosis was confirmed. At that moment Amy realized that she was a cancer patient.

Being a mom and fighting cancer too gave Amy little time for self-pity. Kelly was three years old and Cody was five, and with every surgery and chemotherapy treatment, she knew that she'd be healthy again. Her friends were a terrific emotional support team and two of them were breast cancer survivors. They knew exactly what Amy needed and buoyed her spirits with phone calls, delivered prepared meals, and even hired a maid to clean her house for six months.

In less than a year, Amy had eight surgeries, including a double mastectomy and reconstruction. Except for a month to rest from the mastectomy very little kept Amy from exercise, her other major passion. During the course of her chemotherapy regime she taught twelve aerobics classes a week and was a personal trainer for several clients. These activities gave normalcy back to Amy's life and fueled a positive attitude that she believes helped her to survive. Exercise helped her heal more quickly too and motivated her to return to the gym.

It's been several years since her surgery, and Amy is cancer-free. She has trained many breast cancer survivors too and when they learn that she's a survivor an instant camaraderie is established. Amy is now a certified Advanced Cancer Exercise Specialist, has raced in six triathlons, is a mom to her children, and is proud to be a cancer survivor.

***

"Two years to live?" Celeste protested in disbelief to her husband Bill. The doctor had called to give them the news that the mole taken off her arm was melanoma.

"I can't die," Celeste protested with tears in her eyes, "I'm only thirty-one years old. What will you and the children do without me?" At the time of her diagnosis her three children were six months, eight, and eleven years old.

Months earlier, her obstetrician was concerned about the mole too, "Celeste, we need to take that mole off, it looks bad."

"Oh, well, after the baby comes, you can take it off. I'm not worried." Her father always called the mole a "tick" because ever since Celeste was a teenager, that's exactly what it looked like. But, during her last pregnancy it grew to the size of a thumbnail. That was in 1961.

With the thought of cancer, Celeste began to cry. She never knew anyone who'd survived the disease and was sure that she'd die too. She cried through her words to her husband, "Why is this happening to me? I don't understand it."

However, Celeste believed in miracles and faith healing. She'd always been a church-going person, but now she had cancer and she cried at the thought that somehow she'd fallen out of favor with God. For weeks, they were held in the waiting room for up to six hours a day just to see the doctor. The mole was removed but further surgery was required to see if the melanoma had spread. The doctor, a leading specialist in melanoma, noticed that she had a suspicious knot on the inside of both knees.

"We'll have to remove those knots, they may be cancerous also," he said. Then, he prepared her for the worst-case scenario, "It's possible that we may have to remove your right arm and both legs."

Celeste's voice wobbled, "What is the best I can expect?"

"If the cancer hasn't spread, we might get by with only partial amputation of your arm and chemotherapy treatment. But, if we get inside and find out that the cancer has spread far along, you might have two years to live at the most."

"Why? Why?" Celeste repeated over and over. What she'd done to make God not favor her she wondered? She had so many plans for her life. She wanted to finish her education after her children were in school and become a teacher. Now, it seemed that life was never going to be the way she intended.

One morning, as she scrambled eggs with her baby on her hip, tears ran down her cheeks and she began to pray. "Lord, I know if you take me to heaven, Bill can find another woman to love him. He is so lovable and wonderful. But, Lord, there is not one woman on this earth that will love these children like I do. If you will heal me so that I can raise my children, I will serve you any way you want me to for the rest of my life."

After surgery, the doctor came to tell Celeste the good news. " I believe you are a miracle lady," he said. "We could not find one cancer cell in your body. We took a six-inch section from your arm and there was no cancer. We removed each knot in your knees, and they were cancer-free too. We are going to watch you to make sure there isn't any more trouble with cancer."

Celeste was cancer-free.

Celeste remembered her promise to God. She volunteered to work at church, was the president of the women's missionary group, led the young adults' Sunday School department, and taught the women in the department, too. Celeste and Bill taught the teenagers on Sunday nights and were at the church nearly every weeknight and weekday.

Celeste continued her education and received teaching certificates in Bilingual Education, Kindergarten, and English as a Second Language. She later became a principal, earned a Masters in Educational Administration with a mid-management certificate then received a Doctorate in Education and served as the Dean of Education and International Students. Celeste taught many young adults to speak English and trained teachers for Christian schools. She also became a mother figure to many of them and an integral part of their lives. Now, in her seventies, a grandmother thirteen times and a great-grandmother too, Celeste writes Christian storybooks for children and is grateful for all of her blessings.

***

Long before Tracy was born, someone told Arvid about the special bond that exists between fathers and daughters. It's now been several years since Tracy's diagnosis, but Arvid will never forget the night when the family first learned that his daughter might be taken from him. He was the Stephen Ministry Leader at his church and during a regular Wednesday night meeting his wife, Ann, came into the classroom with an urgent look on her face. Out in the hall, Ann's eyes were stern as she reached for her husband's hand. Arvid's eyes filled with tears in anticipation. Over and over, the word cancer was used. Arvid couldn't believe it. Not Tracy. Not my beautiful Tracy, he thought. From the moment of her birth, she was perfect and he vowed to protect her from harm.

Cancer had already knocked on the family's door. Ann's mother had colon cancer and Arvid's grandfather had stomach cancer. Ann continued to give the news and thoughts raced through Arvid's head. Maybe there was a misdiagnosis, or even a confusion of names with tests results, he thought. Finally, Ann stopped talking and he didn't know what to do or say. He walked back into the classroom, looked at everyone in shock and sat down, unable to speak. Within moments, he was surrounded by a group of caring, loving, and compassionate men and women who prayed with him.

"Fathers have interesting roles, often misunderstood and dictated by society. As I drove home from church that evening, I knew that I would need to be the strong one in our family. Tracy's siblings love her very much and would be devastated with the news. Ann, too, is always one to be emotional when something terrible like this happens to our family. My role has always been to help us stay the course, to be logical and rational, and not to dwell on the dark side. Our family needed balance and I decided to be the counterweight when things got too difficult during Tracy's cancer battle."

As Arvid drove home and into the driveway, he reflected on how different all of their lives were as compared to just a few hours earlier. It was illogical. It was unfair. Tracy was only twenty-eight years old with a newborn infant and a toddler. Arvid felt powerless to protect, or to fix the problem, as he had always done for his family. As a father, he wasn't sure of his role in this new situation because Tracy was a married woman. How could he guide and protect her without stepping over the boundaries of her marriage and adult life? For a while, Arvid felt like a helpless observer and he prayed that God and Tracy's doctors would provide her with the greatest amount of help. Soon he found his place in the crisis and helped with the children in ways that would work for Tracy and her husband. He drove Tracy once a week to radiation therapy and this became their special time together.

"I'd carefully select a CD for each trip and we'd listen to encouraging music. I'd fight back tears on each trip to the hospital as I watched my little girl be brave for us all. By this time, Tracy had already lost her voice due to radiation and was using a 'magic pad' to communicate with me. I'd read her responses and deep within her gaze she'd imploringly ask me if everything was going to be all right. I'd nod back and always remained strong and positive for her."

As the crisis wore on, Tracy's cancer diagnosis left Arvid emotionally numb. He felt unable to get in touch with himself. He'd set his fears and pains aside in order to be a man of action for his family. Logically, he knew that it was unhealthy to ignore his feelings, but for all of his training as a minister and counselor, he couldn't seem to help himself.

"I desperately needed to cry and let go of all the emotions welling up inside me. The time was never right, the place was never right and instead I'd hold everything inside until I felt like I'd burst. My social education taught me that it was my duty to be a strong man in difficult situations. My religious faith taught me to be unwavering in my devotion, no matter what. But a building resentment was growing deep inside me. I resented the fact this was happening again in our family and to our youngest daughter. I felt powerless as the protector of my family. People had a say in our lives now, as well-intended church members came up to me and made suggestions about where Tracy should be receiving care. They warned that we had only one chance to get her well or that such and such institution is the only place to receive cancer treatment. The pressure was mounting within me and had nowhere to go."

Tracy's radiation therapy spanned six weeks. Sleep was difficult for Arvid during that time and he felt separated from God. As he held Tracy's children one day, he wondered if they'd ever hear their mother's voice again, or how their lives would be if Tracy died. How will I explain her death to them and why God took their mother away, he wondered? One stormy afternoon, he stared out the living room window as thunder and lightning raged across the sky. Arvid's thoughts pooled about all the suffering in his family because of cancer. How can I possibly endure the pain and loss of Tracy if she isn't cured, he wondered. With these thoughts, his anger soared. He had to get away. Immediately, he packed an overnight bag and told his wife that he needed to leave in order to think. Ann understood and asked that he call her when he was ready to talk. Arvid didn't know where he was going but knew that he needed to leave Dallas and find space enough to breathe.

The next thing he knew, a road sign indicated Austin city limits.

Once in his hotel, he collapsed into a chair and all the pent up emotions freely poured.

"I spent the entire night looking out my window at the pouring rain and powerful winds and cried my tears of pain, fear, sorrow, and frustration until I couldn't any longer," he said.

Tracy's cancer battle is over and life is back to normal. Though time has passed, it's sometimes still hard for Arvid to talk or even write about that time in his life without experiencing fear and a sense of helplessness. Prayer provides the comfort that he needs when life's answers are uncertain. Tracy is healthy and life is happy again.

***

So, though my energy levels had drastically diminished and my complexion was akin to ghost-white due to anemia, I continued to go to work throughout the first six months of chemotherapy. Texas heat mixed with the side effects of menopause forced me to switch to hats instead of wigs for a while. One day, a co-worker who knew me well came to say that she'd overheard a group of new employees gossip about the person who wore hats every day. "Does she think she's special or something? Who does she think she is?" said one person.

"Either that, or maybe she has a lot of really bad hair days," said another and they all laughed. This group of gossipers was hired while I was hospitalized for the Staph infection and didn't know me at all. My "informant" co-worker let this group know that the person they gossiped and laughed about had cancer and that was the reason for the hats. Their mouths popped open at this news and according to her there was never a more embarrassed, or speechless group of people. She was angry about the incident and was troubled by the injustice. She felt embarrassed and tried to protect me from their cruelty. I thanked her for her thoughtful consideration but chances were that I never would have known about the incident at all if she didn't tell me and I wasn't sure that I was better off for the knowledge. Anytime I saw one of them afterward, I was forced to endure their pathetic, wide-eyed looks of pity.

Having to conceal the fact that I had cancer under stylish wigs, make-up and restrictive clothing just to meet a societal standard irritated my sensibilities. Had I been a man, my appearance would hardly have mattered to anyone, but for whatever reason, people need to see a woman with hair in order to be right with the world.

Another incident at work was particularly strange and to this day I'm unclear about the interest and motivation of two "vultures" that visited my desk. I do know for certain that I felt ganged up on. I was married just a few weeks and two framed wedding pictures proudly sat on my desk.

"What does your husband think?" one woman asked.

"Think about what?" I replied with feigned ignorance. I knew that she meant my cancer diagnosis, but I wouldn't give her the benefit of an assumed understanding, as though cancer were the entirety of my life. Besides I wanted to hear her say the word cancer. None of them did. "What is he supposed to think?" I asked back.

"Is he going to stick around?" another asked. They knew that I was a newlywed and the abrupt callousness of that question was as harsh as any chemotherapy cocktail.

"Why wouldn't he? He's my husband," I returned.

"I can't believe he married you anyway," said another. I wasn't sure if that was a compliment or an insult, but it didn't feel good.

"Why are you shocked that a man who loves me would marry me?" I questioned. "Am I somehow not worthy of love and happiness because I have cancer?" I asked them. They stuttered in surprise of my question.

"What you need to do is to ask whether your own husbands would do the same," I said. "I'm lucky, I don't have to waste twenty five years to find out that my marriage vows are worthless and my husband is a jerk. I sure hope that you don't have to." I gave an ambiguous smile and there was silence as they picked their jaws up off the floor and left.

How dare they attempt to cast darkness on the one beautiful and secure thing that I had in my life? To them, a cancer diagnosis meant that you lost everything, even love, because you were not worthy of it any longer. I felt sad for them. Though I had cancer, I was secure in love, happy, more confident than ever and the vultures didn't get the coffee break soap opera they expected.

I marched into Laura's office to inform her of my "vulturous" encounter and also let her know that I'd put into practice all of the previous discussions we'd had about balance and boundaries. I wouldn't be tolerant of further verbal abuse while on the job.

I was the first cancer case the office had ever encountered and there was nothing in the rulebook under "employee interactions with a co-worker on chemo."

"How do you plan to protect me from this type of behavior in the future?" I asked Laura. She wasn't sure how, or if she could protect me, but she did her best and I was always grateful for her support. It remained a delicate gray area where disciplinary action was concerned, but when diplomacy failed and motives were unclear, I protected myself and found that people understood my boundaries better when I rammed against theirs. We decided to attribute the rudeness of the vultures to pure ignorance. Through clenched teeth, I let it slide. Laura and I laughed and went back to work.

Here and there I was still lucky enough to catch a few energy spurts and managed a once-a-week workout with exhausted efforts. I probably could've continued this for a while longer if I had only kept my big mouth shut. I bounced into Dr. Smith's office for chemotherapy one day all sweaty and still pumped from a workout session. My journal entry says it all.

August 3, 2000

Dr. Smith asked me how I was handling the chemotherapy. "Oh, great," I said, "I just finished a nine-mile bike ride at the gym." He was astonished. I flexed my bicep to show off, laughed and said, "Chemo can't keep me down." The doctor was pleased to learn of my progress and said that he now wanted to be more aggressive against my cancer in the last two months of treatment. He turned to the nurse and said, "Let's increase her chemo dosage, I think she can handle it." I wanted to take back all my boasts and brags but it was too late, there were witnesses. And now I have to take my medicine. More chemo please!

***

So, now with a heavy chemo load and still having to deal with the stupidity of co-workers who didn't understand the meaning of hope and challenged the integrity of my medical decisions, I felt saddled with more adversity. Desk-side visits now included chats about alternative methods that might cure me of cancer though they had absolutely no knowledge about what they discussed. Instead, they referred to what they had heard third-hand, read on the front cover of a magazine, or had heard in a fifteen-second teaser on the news about the latest speculative hope of some research study.

I'm sure if in the same situation, these co-workers wouldn't have followed their own advice. Though some people claim to have been healed with holistic approaches such as acupuncture, massage, chiropractic, colonics, oxygen baths, yoga, meditation, aromatherapy, barley green, medicinal mushrooms, macrobiotic diet, eat for your blood type diet, and a long list of other alternatives; none of these approaches are proven by the scientific community as an effective treatment to prevent or cure cancer. Until science produces a cure for all cancers, oncology remains an inexact science though others with a more hopeful view like to say, 'a science in pursuit of answers.' No matter your viewpoint, either spin, taken down to its common denominator provides the same scary outcome for you and me—despite billions of dollars spent on research there is still no cure for cancer.

Alternative therapies can improve a patient's quality of life by reducing nausea, assisting pain management, boosting the immune system, or lowering stress. Holistic therapies do not cure cancer and no scientific data can support that claim. Yet, it was easy for some people to look me in the face, unknowledgeable and content of their clean bill of health, while they criticized my life and death decisions. All things considered, my responses were calm, straight-faced, and quite diplomatic. On numerous occasions I felt held hostage by the protocol and politics of the work environment which didn't allow me the freedom to say what I really thought of my co-workers' rudeness and ignorance, but I continued to make sure that management knew.

So, while the normalcy of a daily work routine was good for my mind, it was evident that I was no longer in a normal situation. The effects of chemo-related fatigue intensified, and one particular day, I woke up at my desk in a puddle of drool. As much as I hated to admit it, chemo had the better of me now.

The work atmosphere continued to prove to be an unstable place for me while I was sick and this was a great disappointment. From an intellectual point of view, I needed the productivity of work, but in contrast, people constantly focused on my hair loss whenever they'd see me as though that's all there was to a cancer battle. Others repeatedly commented on how "normal" I looked, which was intended to be a compliment, but the inference was clear that I was now abnormal.

One person suggested that a strong cup of coffee might help against my chemo-related fatigue. I wished he were in my shoes for five minutes so that he'd know the limited powers of a double espresso. Though some of my co-workers were jerks, management was terrific. I got a call one day that the department Director wanted to interview me for the position I applied for before my diagnosis. I was thrilled to still be a contender and wanted to skip through the hallways and sing, "I Will Survive," but ten seconds into my victory, reality kicked in. I was really sick. When I met with the Director to discuss the position she explained that there'd be travel, people to manage and it would be fast-paced. She'd seen me in action plenty of times before and didn't doubt my ability even though I'd been on chemo for a couple of months.

"Do you think you're up for the challenge?" she asked me.

One side of my brain screamed, Yes! And the other said, No! Six months earlier, I would've dove into murky, deep waters filled with sharks and alligators for this opportunity to have this position, but my life had changed in six months. I didn't want to accept the job if I couldn't succeed with high marks.

"I can't believe that I'm about to say this, but I think I'll have to pass," I told the department Director. "I wanted this position so much. But my health is too unpredictable right now for me to commit to anything new. I wouldn't want to fail and affect the progress of the entire department."

She understood and conveyed her sorrow and support for my cancer battle. She told me that I was well liked by management and assured me that when I was ready, the opportunity to climb the corporate ladder would be there for me. My department Director gave me new confidence that day and in a way, I already felt promoted.

The decline of my health due to continuous chemo and two more incidents at work confirmed that it was time for me to stay home and tend to my illness. One day, as I exited a bathroom stall, a co-worker who I hardly knew, abruptly asked me if I'd be able to have children since I had cancer, and if I couldn't, would my husband divorce me. My body clenched with anger and embarrassment to have my private life and hopes strewn about the bathroom. With her comment, I not only felt humiliated for myself but also envisioned the progress of a hundred years of women's rights slide into a canyon of eternal ignorance. I was raised in a generation that taught girls that they could be anything: an astronaut, the president of a company, even the President of the United States. My co-worker's comment reminded me that regardless of education levels, professional accomplishments, or personal goals, many people still believe that a woman's value is measured by the integrity of her womb. I hid my offended expression while I washed my hands, re-adjusted my bra straps out of sight, and checked my lipstick. The other people in the bathroom pretended not to hear. I gave some general reply and then went directly to Laura's office to inform her of what had just happened. It was difficult to hold my head up every day when people knowingly or not sought to strike me down with rude comments and innuendo. I felt assaulted by the bathroom incident and my nostrils flared like a bull as I described the scene to Laura.

"She said what? In the bathroom?" It all sounded so hilarious now as Laura scrunched up her face in disbelief and her mouth fell open in an attempt to picture the scene.

"Yup," I said, "as I came out of the stall." By the second retelling, Laura and I were unable to do more than hold our stomachs with laughter from the ridiculousness of that and the hundred other things that had been said to me since my diagnosis.

However, a final incident at work convinced me that it was time to stay home for a while and rest. A co-worker who was one of the vultures came by my desk and said that she'd been thinking of me. For a moment, I thought that perhaps she'd attended a sensitivity course, but she gave a strange laugh and said that she owed thanks to God that a recent lump found under her arm was benign. She went on and on about her relationship with God, and how her pastor had prayed with her. After she shared the story of her cancer scare, she trotted off to her desk and the certainties of her life. Many times, I'd seen her amid the haze of the smoker's hovel outside as she and others puffed away during a fifteen-minute break in any kind of weather just to have their carcinogenic fix.

I had prayed to God, too. Why did God listen to her prayers and not mine? Was her life more valuable? Was it possible that God didn't love me? As I sat in front of my computer, I felt unable to move and could only stare at the blurred numbers on the spreadsheet in front of me. Fifty thousand thoughts converged into one big mess. I couldn't permit my personal integrity, hopes, and spiritual faith to be jeopardized on someone's coffee break any longer. I didn't return to work until the following spring after radiation treatment was over.

***

The experience of cancer has allowed me to step back, take stock, and do the difficult work of cleaning out the closet of my life. Thank goodness, I was never in the habit of being a pack rat. I'd throw something out if I didn't see a use for it in five years. In terms of a life with cancer, I've used the same principles. If a choice were possible, I'd no longer place myself among people or situations that induced stress or anxiety. My goal was to achieve a better balance. It wasn't difficult anymore to let go of unhealthy relationships especially when I equated them to a disease.

Survival from cancer is my life-long goal and anyone who can't or won't understand is a part of the problem and not the solution. While the majority have supported my efforts towards renewed health, some never seemed to understand, or preferred to be in denial about how sick I was. In one such instance, that person was a relative who really should have known better, but for whom I was less than surprised for his commentary about my selfishness. I'd been on chemo for several months and expressed to this person that I had to put my health needs first and would be unable to fly to New York in order to attend a family event.

"Don't you think you're being kind of selfish?" he questioned.

I hadn't been acquainted with this level of lunatic logic. To a person with cancer being selfless might mean death. In an instant, I remembered the time when a nurse reprimanded me for not reporting my 101 degree fever, but I didn't want to bother the doctor, I told her.

"Get that thought right out of your head and don't you ever do that again," she said with a low rumble in her voice that made me take notice. "A fever means infection and for you right now, that could be life threatening." She looked really pissed off at me. I felt horrible for making her mad.

In my former days, a low-grade fever was something that I toughed through and now I was to treat it with life urgency. I'd been raised with the idea that doctors were very important and busy people. I had never called a doctor in the middle of the night for anything, especially not a low-grade fever, I explained to her.

"I don't care what time it is, you call the doctor," she said a few octaves higher. "You have cancer, Michelle. So, if there's ever a time to be selfish, it is right now."

It kind of stung my conscious to be reminded of the fact that I had cancer, but I didn't want to die because of my sheer stupidity either. I wised up.

The effects of chemo are cumulative, though many are temporary. Once chemo ends and a body can recover, most side effects disappear. The longer I took chemo the more issues I had: numbness in my limbs, dizziness, fatigue, lack of balance, bruising, shortness of breath, and many others.

Chemo-related fatigue was the most difficult of all the side effects and is still a daily issue for me, though not as intense as when I was in treatment. During chemo, a lack of concentration was also another temporary side effect that made a simple task like reading more difficult. Reading has always been as effortless as breathing for me and because of my years in academic pursuits, I was in a regular routine of reading volumes and writing research papers. The effects of chemotherapy slowed my pace a bit and one evening while studying, I read the same line over and over and still didn't know what it meant. I adjusted to the pace, and reminded myself that not only was it a temporary condition, but the achievement of a job well done is more important than the pace in which it is achieved.

***

Joey and I enjoy going to the movie theater together, but chemo-related fatigue, forgetfulness and a lack of concentration made going to the movies a totally different experience. The crowds, the loud sounds, the heavy perfume on the lady in front, or in back of me gave me a headache. The effort to climb to the upper balcony for a good seat exhausted me. On a few occasions, I fell asleep as the mega watt sound of explosions and blood curdling screams shook the theater, but could not rouse me from my slumber. On those occasions when I didn't fall asleep, I was often unable to follow the details of the plot, especially a mystery where the slightest word or gesture provided needed clues for the big reveal at the end. I'd whisper a hundred questions to Joey.

"Hey, I don't get it. How come he's doing that?" Joey would explain to me in Morse code-like sentences what had happened three scenes earlier.

"Don't you remember...when he saw that guy...the one with the briefcase...talking to that lady...the one with the foreign accent?..."

We'd go back and forth until I'd realize that I had no idea what was going on and just stopped asking questions. I'm sure we annoyed everyone else around us too. I didn't want to go to the movies anymore. I shared my thoughts and feelings with Joey and was happy to know that he understood this too. So, we made adjustments and soon our movie night-out switched to our upstairs home theater.

"What do you want to watch tonight?" Joey would ask me.

"Something that doesn't require a lot of thought, how about a comedy," I'd say. The Three Stooges and re-runs of Cheers, and I Love Lucy were always favorites and sometimes we'd get a little silly around the house just out of the blue and imitate the goofiness of the Stooges with fake nose pulls and eye pokes at one another as we'd say things like: "Swointenly," "Nyuck-Nyuck," and "Why, I oughta…Boink!"

Throughout my illness, Joey and I made conscious efforts to add comfort and beauty to our home with ordinary things: soft pillows, plush towels and blankets, and scented candles. These everyday things I'd once taken for granted, now mattered to my quality of life and helped me cope through a day. Every day was special for us; hugs, kisses, and "I love you" were in supply.

Of course, we did a fair share of venting to one another too mostly at the situation itself, which helped to get out all the frustrations and redirected us back to the goal, which was to be healthy again. On some days, I was so sick that escape and denial were preferable to the efforts of creative coping strategies.

Now that I wasn't at work anymore, I tried to have days when the word cancer wasn't used at all. I just wanted to be normal again. I couldn't control the fact that I had cancer. I couldn't always control the side effects of cancer treatments either, but I could, and did control my perception and behavior within the situation, and in doing so, I felt empowered in my new normal. Joey and I chose to be positive and found a multitude of tactics that helped lift our mood when the roadblocks of cancer were thrown in our path. Some of my coping strategies might seem a little kooky, but the situation of a long illness required creativity when I couldn't leave the house for days and weeks.

On days that my mood was low, I wore my good jewelry just to feel pretty around the house. I lit a scented candle, cuddled with my favorite fuzzy blanket, and listened to music that brought back good memories. When the level of my white blood didn't put me at risk for infection, I picked bouquets of flowers from my garden and arranged them in vases throughout the house so that everywhere I looked there was a splash of color and vitality. Other strategies had the power to lift my spirits too, and helped me get through some really bad days. For example, I ate from the good china, used cloth napkins instead of paper, and drank from the crystal. I figured, why wait for a special occasion, when every day was special and might be my last. On days when I looked as terrible as I felt, a little lipstick and a colorful scarf tied around my neck had the ability to perk me up and take the pallor out of my complexion and the dullness out of my eyes. On good days when my energy was up and my blood counts, too, I'd make a date with myself to bask in the glory of being out in the world. I felt great to just be alive and wasn't waiting to be cured in order to live.

***

Joey and I planned for the future and that future included children. We hoped to have at least one child and discussed all of the joys and hard work that parenthood would bring. We'd smile in anticipation of family vacations to the mountain resorts of New York, the beaches of Florida and Disney World, the Caribbean islands, or historical destinations throughout Europe. We talked about the many things we'd teach our child and the opportunities we'd offer: the arts, science, foreign language, music and especially the experiences of many types of people and humanitarian causes. We'd teach the traditions, establish new ones of our own and with great joy, celebrate holidays, and birthdays. We laughed and acted out how we'd look and sound thirty years from now and imagined the stories we'd tell our grandchildren around the Sunday dinner table of how we met and fell in love. Joey and I had plans to last for many decades and as a result, I had plenty of reasons to say goodbye to cancer.

Dr. Smith wasn't kidding when he said that he was "turning up the chemo." The increased dosage was oppressive. Between Joey's work schedule and my lack of energy, we hired a housekeeper and I now did the grocery shopping through an on-line delivery service. For the sake of my sanity and because I refused to be undermined by cancer, I began Graduate school in August and took two courses that fall semester, which required me to attend classes twice a week.

One day as I walked across the campus with a group of fellow classmates, I took one step for every three of theirs. They never knew that I had cancer and most of my professors didn't know either unless I told them. The university was a place where I felt safe and free. Within the atmosphere of academics, my cancer battle wasn't everyone's business. My opinions mattered and weren't weighted with public fears and sentiments about cancer.

By September, the increased dosage of chemo made me sleep sometimes fifteen hours at a time. My energy was sparse and sleep patterns were unpredictable. When I was awake, I'd study and prepare for class no matter if it was 2:00 a.m. The responsibility of Graduate classes twice a week forced me to be disciplined when I had no energy. The fact that I no longer had a job to go to every day made me a little depressed. On some days, I felt like a big loser especially when I couldn't climb to the second floor of my house. But, I'd remember that it wasn't my will, it was my health that declined.

My weekly workouts were now physically impossible, but like everything else, I tried to compensate for this too. With an eight-pound barbell and five-pound ankle weights, I did bicep curls and leg lifts in front of the living room television just to keep my body in motion. My friends reminded me that "muscle had memory," and I hoped the expression was true. I longed for the old days of back-to-back aerobics classes and deep squats with one hundred and fifty pound weights on my shoulders. I longed for the days when I wouldn't stagger across the room for a glass of water. I'd be back again, I told myself, and would be stronger than ever.

Joey continued to work his usual long hours and remained just a phone call and a short distance from home. We'd made a pact to maintain normalcy as much as possible, but on many days he just wanted to stay home with me. I'd tell him that I was fine and that I'd call him if needed. There were a few days that I had to plead with him to go to work and nudge him out the door. I was sick, but far from incapacitated. For me to cope within the chaos of cancer, I needed to be as independent as possible and didn't want anyone to hold my hand or wait on me like I was helpless.

Not only had my chemo been increased, but anticipatory nausea took hold of me, which was a bizarre phenomenon that was thankfully temporary. Like clockwork, as each chemo date approached, I was unable to control the anxiety that set in. Heart palpitations and nausea were routine. The knowledge of being poisoned was more intense than my logic. My body convulsed and uncontrollable tears fell in anticipation of the chemo assault that I was about to encounter.

Before Joey and I walked into the cancer center, I'd take a few deep breaths to psyche myself up and imagined myself a soldier ready to race across the battlefield. Without fail, as soon as the cancer center's electric double doors swung open, I wanted to gag. Everything about the cancer center now made me ill: the voice of the receptionist, the smell of alcohol wipes, the air freshener in the bathroom and even the sight of people who were now my friends.

A few months earlier, I didn't know the meaning of the word oncology and now I had too much information and hated that I did. I knew the difference between a butterfly needle and one adequate for CT scans. The track marks on my arms told me which veins were good prospects for regular blood draws and my vocabulary included words like: Cytoxan, Vincristine, Etoposide and other drugs. I cringed one day as I approached the chemo room and as Dr. Smith passed by he casually asked, "How are you doing?"

I exploded. "I'm tired of this!" Already in a heightened state of emotion from the anticipatory condition on the drive over, I vented my frustrations to the doctor: "I don't look or feel like myself, I'm hot flashing every twenty minutes. I can't work out anymore and I can't fit into my new leather pants."

He nodded as I spewed out my list of grievances.

"Worst of all, no matter how hard I try, I can't fall asleep and I'm up until four a.m., watching Gilligan's Island." The steroids were responsible for that side effect. Mild sleeping pills were prescribed but I refused to take them.

"I can't take much more of this crap!" I told Dr. Smith about the anticipatory nausea I suffered. "I can't do this anymore," I said. "You'll have to knock me out with drugs for the rest of these chemo sessions because I can't deal with it. By the time I get to your office I'm a wreck. I just want to sleep through the treatments so just knock me out on arrival," I said.

"No problem," said Dr. Smith, "we can do that. Chemo is almost over, you've come this far, you can do it." We discussed other ways to combat my anticipatory nausea like with the scent of vanilla, creative visualization, and even changing the location of my treatment. I felt more confident with the knowledge that Dr. Smith believed in me and also realized that I should've communicated my feelings much earlier.

By October, Dr. Smith had great news for us. The tumor in my chest was gone. Six weeks of radiation would follow it up to be sure that every last cell was killed.

"Don't take it personally, Dr. Smith, but I'm not coming back here ever again. Can you give me two more months of chemo?" He was shocked to hear me volunteer for more.

"What about all the anticipatory issues?"

"I'll just tell myself to get over it. I'm through with cancer," I said. "If six months of chemo made the tumor disappear, then two more months will be even better." I needed to be an over-achiever in this if only to know that the enemy was decapitated, without limbs, disemboweled, and bludgeoned with such a maniacal force that it would never rise up to get me again like some boogeyman-monster under my bed.

"I have to go the distance with this," I said to the doctor. "I need to know that I did everything possible and went beyond what was asked of me."

The doctor understood. Thankfully, the additional chemo fit into an acceptable medical protocol too. So, I willingly suffered through two more months in the hope that I'd be cancer-free. Along with my determination to destroy cancer for good, my bouts with anticipatory nausea left as mysteriously as they came. Though I still had weeks of radiation ahead of me, I felt positive that I'd won my battle against cancer.

By late November, my chemo was in high gear and so was my schoolwork. Physically and mentally, I'd never worked so hard and I finished the semester with perfect grades. During a final exam in December, fever raged and the area around my medi-port ached. This time, I knew that it was another Staph infection. The port was removed and the area was so badly infected that it couldn't be stitched shut. I had an open wound in my chest about the size of a quarter and several inches deep, which Joey would end up packing and re-packing twice a day. In previous months of feeling helpless about my illness, Joey now felt that he could do something to help me besides just being an understanding husband and handing me tissues.

As a patient, I was given a schedule of medicines and with it I had a plan of action, but a caregiver is given no set of instructions and often struggles to know the best way to help. As my caregiver, Joey's responsibilities were all encompassing. At home and elsewhere he had to know it all and follow through when I was too sick to speak for myself. He knew all appointment times and everything pertaining to my medicines just about better than I did. When I'd forget that Finergin and Benadryl gave me "jumpy legs," Joey knew better and then another medicine would be prescribed. He developed a rapport with the medical staff and learned his way around the hospital like it was our second home. In these ways, he helped us both through the process.

So, with pus oozing from a hole in my chest, the process of changing the gauze was too painful for me to do. As vile as it was, it was an important role for Joey and he seemed to glow with his newly won task. I was never more grossed out as I watched him pull out green and yellow pus-soaked strips of gauze, then repack the wound with fresh new gauze to soak up the rest of the pus. As the pus was removed daily, the hole slowly closed and healed after a month.

That New Year's Eve, we braved a rare Texas snowstorm just to have sushi and came home in time to toast 2001 with Dick Clark in Times Square on television. Despite the difficulties of 2000, the year was also a happy one for us. We were married, had a home, Joey was steadily employed, and we had health benefits. We were grateful and knew that it was more than a lot of people had. Most of all, we had each other and that was everything. The next part in my journey towards a cancer-free life was radiation treatments that were soon to begin.

***

February 12, 2001

So far I've completed 1 month of radiation to the throat and chest area. I have about 2 weeks more to go. I am so tired all the time and am having difficulty breathing and swallowing. My internal tissue is swollen like I've been cooked. I feel like I'm choking all the time and can't sleep at night because of it. Dr. Gilbert said that after treatments are over the healing process would begin and could take up to a year. Ten months of drugs has killed the tumor but has destroyed healthy cells too. I am so tired.

***

Despite what everyone told me about radiation treatment being "a breeze," that wasn't the case for me. I was told that most people experience radiation side-effects weeks after treatment, but mine were immediate. The first humiliation was laying bare-breasted with magic marker dots from neck to diaphragm as two strangers positioned me over the scan. Once positioned, I had to remain still as they'd leave the room to turn the switch like an executioner. In those few seconds, I felt very alone as radiation surged through me. I'd smell faint fumes, and my saliva tasted like metal as healthy internal tissue and blood were destroyed along with any cancer cells that might still lurk about. Radiation treatments every day for six weeks produced raw, burnt flesh that throbbed with pain and itched as if a thousand red fire ants gnawed at me. Two years later, I still felt the phantom fire ants on my back, especially when I'd sweat. In the meantime, to relieve my radiation burns, I'd slather aloe on a piece of plastic and lay in the cool relief.

There, in my wallow of aloe, I'd think about how proud I'd feel with my name inscribed on The Cancer Monument's granite walls, surrounded by the courageous names of thousands who had also battled cancer. I'd imagine myself sitting by the monument's peaceful fountains with my child one day, as I'd explain how the 60,000 Honoree names had come to be there. As the years passed by, we'd take notice of how large the four trees that marked each symbolic point of entry had grown, and we'd welcome thousands of people from across the land. I'd imagine that Joey and I would stop by the monument on our way to one of our special Sunday outings. There at the monument site, we'd see families stand before the great granite walls in search of names. They'd lay an offering of flowers, a poem, letter or teddy bear and the process of healing grief and living life would be made easier. As I lay in my pool of aloe, I'd feel renewed with hope for the future.

I hoped that Joey and I would come to know the stories of many valiant cancer heroes and their families. I'd proclaim, "You have each made this possible by inscribing the names of your honored Heroes on these granite walls. This is your monument." These thoughts and many more spurred me on in my quest for health.

I knew what The Cancer Monument meant to me and hoped that it would mean that, and more to others. I envisioned it every day, but still wasn't quite sure of how to bring it to the public. There were no footsteps to follow in. It had never been done before. Somehow the idea that resided in my head and on paper would have to become a full-blown national campaign.

My radiation treatments were over and Dr. Gilbert told me the good news: The scans showed no evidence of cancer. I was pronounced as being in remission.

"You're cancer-free," said Dr. Gilbert, "go live a normal, happy life."

I didn't know what to say and didn't know what normal was anymore. "How do I live a normal life now?" I asked. I couldn't go back to the old normal because I'd changed so much in a year.

"Go back to what you did before you had cancer and just take things one day at a time," he said.

Maybe this was normal. It was certainly my normal and maybe that was all that mattered anyway. A cancer-free existence required more preparation than I ever expected. The words "you're cured" didn't prompt a scene of me skipping out of the cancer center with a song on my lips to meet the glorious day. I drove home with a heavy mind filled with questions. I could now identify with the caged animal who knows nothing but captivity; though unknown freedoms tempt from just a few feet away the animal does not venture beyond the security of the cage.

I figured that a return to work was about as close to normal as I could get so I called Laura and planned my return in May. Included in the freedom from cancer, was a strange feeling that alarmed and stunned me. I felt guilty for being alive.

<u>March 9, 2001</u>

Sometimes I feel guilty for being a survivor. I've heard of survivor's guilt but I didn't understand it until now. I thought that I'd be swinging from chandeliers to be cancer-free, but there are times when I wonder why I was spared instead of a mother of three. What is really the grand purpose of my existence in this world that so requires my participation? Thankfully, this new survivor's guilt isn't constant. It comes in the quiet times of my mind and yet other times it is not on my mind at all. When I take a walk and feel the wind on my face or make a nice dinner for Joey, I am so grateful and proud for the chance to live again. So far, I am walking away from cancer intact. I have not been disfigured, lost limbs, or organs to this disease, unlike so many others. I will have to work through these strange and unhealthy feelings of survivor's guilt.

***

The spring of 2001 brought a strange mixture of thoughts and feelings for me. The joy of newly sprung hair allowed me to put away my hats and wigs but this victory overlapped with bizarre bouts of survivor's guilt and new boundary-setting issues. One day as I stood in the grocery store checkout line, I fanned through the pages of a fashion magazine. So, this is what I'm supposed to look like this season, I chuckled to myself. At that moment a woman came up behind me and said, "Oh, I just love your hair!"

***

Also during that spring, I met with a local newspaper editor to discuss an idea that I had for a regular column about cancer. My column was called "Surviving Cancer" and provided insight into many areas that are a part of the cancer journey. I was thrilled and grateful to my editor, Chuck Bloom, for giving me the opportunity and was further validated by the email responses from my readers. I now knew that there were many people who felt as I did about cancer. I wasn't alone. When I gave back to the cause through my column, I felt awesome, and these feelings of belonging and purpose took hold and replaced survivor's guilt. I was a part of a large cancer community that celebrated life, acknowledged and grieved loss, lived for tomorrow, searched for answers, demanded a cure, and was in need of more.

If I'm not alone in the issues that I face, I thought one day, then maybe I'm on target with my monument idea too. I hadn't really done much about the monument beyond my written outlines and sketches. I was still too afraid to take the next step into the unknown. Maybe no one really wanted a cancer monument anyway, I thought. Would it be worth the attempt? Or, should I just focus my energies on my own recovery and life? I wasn't sure of what to do.

Joey and I left for a short vacation to Mexico. There, deep within the jungles, we explored the great and mysterious limestone Mayan temples and pyramids at Chichen Itza and Tulum. Standing in front of those ancient wonders, built with simple stone tools, made my modern-day inspiration for a granite, cancer monument seem more possible. Exhausted from the heat and chemo-related fatigue, I rested under a tree while Joey explored the ruins and climbed to the top of the great temple as though he were Indiana Jones. I'll bet they had cancer too, I thought as I imagined ancient Mayan people living, working, and worshipping the sun.

As we got ready to leave the archaeological site, dark thunderclouds rolled in and blanketed the ancient city in a showy display. Amid the rumble, I felt great to be alive, although vulnerable against the forces of nature. I also realized that in the span of time and the history of the world, as a single human being, I was barely more than a walk-on role…a bit player in a much greater show. However, many people working together for a common goal can leave their mark on history. As we drove away I thought, "If they could clear a jungle two thousand years ago and build a city with no technology, then I can build a cancer monument." But just as no one builds a city alone, so it is with The Cancer Monument.

Upon my return from Mexico, I received a phone call from one of my readers, a woman named Grace, who had been recently diagnosed with lung cancer and was in need of a support group. Grace never smoked so the diagnosis came as quite a shock. She was in her seventies and because of chemo side effects she had difficulty traveling to remote cancer support group meetings. Grace needed a local support group, but there wasn't one. She called me to ask if I would organize a group. But what did I know about support groups when I'd never even been to one? I offered her a few suggestions and gave her some phone numbers to call.

But Grace was a very spiritual woman and said that God spoke to her heart when she read my column in the newspaper and that I was the answer to her prayer. From the flattery perspective, how in the world could I possibly refuse her after that? She had faith in my ability. She saw me as a leader. I was surprised by her assessment, but having a few decades on me in age, I thought perhaps Grace saw qualities in me that I didn't. But beyond the needs of my ego, the bottom line was that I simply couldn't refuse Grace in her great time of need. So, with the help of the American Cancer Society and a local hospital, the first dialogue support group began and continues to serve the needs of the community to this day. I didn't know it then, but Grace had only a year left of life, yet we began a friendship for a lifetime.

I continued to write the newspaper column, helped to facilitate the support group, attended graduate school, and returned to work where I was promoted to a newly created management position. I was finding my new normal. My menstrual cycles attempted a return too and I was under the care of a fertility specialist. Joey and I were thrilled to have cancer behind us and hoped that with a year of recovery I'd be back in shape and ready to start a family.

In the meantime, I struggled with daily fatigue, which made work difficult. My manager, Laura, always understood and encouraged me onward when I thought that my quick return to corporate life was a bad idea. Day after day, as I'd sit at my computer, thoughts of the monument flashed and distracted me from my work as if to say, "Don't forget!" Fear held me back from taking the next step. What if no one wanted the monument? Could 60,000 Honoree names be obtained in a reasonable time frame? What if failure was written in red across my resume as a consequence of my attempt? Where would I construct such a monument?

There were many unanswered questions, but one day I talked to Laura about the monument for the very first time. As I spoke, she was overcome with emotion and tears. I had no picture or website to show her that day, only my conviction, but that alone was enough. She'd always believed in me and her confidence that day convinced me that I followed the right path. To test market the monument, I began to pitch my idea across many states and to a variety of people: cancer survivors, nurses, doctors, community leaders, neighbors, teachers, and other co-workers. All were beyond words, choked with emotion, and though I still had no formal pictures of the monument, everyone could envision the structure as they listened to my ideas. Each person gave me the resounding affirmation that I needed to go forward and finally to a point that it became self-evident; The Cancer Monument was wanted and needed across many public sectors and throughout the country. I talked to my editor, Chuck, about the monument too when I delivered my next column.

He thought that the monument was a great idea and gave me some good advice, "If you want it to be built the way you've envisioned it, you'll have to be the leader all the way."

A part of me just wanted to recover from cancer, live a serene, uneventful life, and spend quiet evenings with Joey. We'd just adopted a Black Labrador Retriever from the animal shelter and wanted to take carefree walks with him. We wanted to work in the garden, growing flowers and herbs, and enjoy our leisurely life. We hadn't planned on a catapult into philanthropy and the responsibilities of public service. But, for over a year, I'd questioned the meaning of normalcy to the point that I now realized that this was my normal. I could never be the person that I was before cancer, nor did I want to be. My cancer journey had forced change, I'd been enlightened on so many levels as a result, and I liked who I'd become. I was thankful to have my blinders removed and now felt more aware and able-bodied than at any other point in my life. I was proud to have battled cancer and was determined to make a difference. The Cancer Monument was the answer and it waited for me to take it to the next level.

I didn't tell everyone the story of how the monument had come to me as a result of prayer, but certain people I knew I could tell. Grace was one of them. Those that knew Grace best said that she "had a direct line to heaven." She believed in The Cancer Monument, was an original Board member, and said that if it were God's will, the monument would be built. When I got discouraged about how slow the wheels of progress moved, she'd remind me that God's time and our time were often very different. I'd remember her words when more stones were thrown in my path however I felt as though I stood on the edge of a cliff. The Cancer Monument had to be brought into public view. I had a choice. I could stand safely on the edge of the cliff and never build The Cancer Monument, or take a step forward into the unknown and trust that public support would be there. The more I thought about it, I realized that the monument's legacy was greater than my fear. More importantly, the people deserved an opportunity to have it. I had to do something.

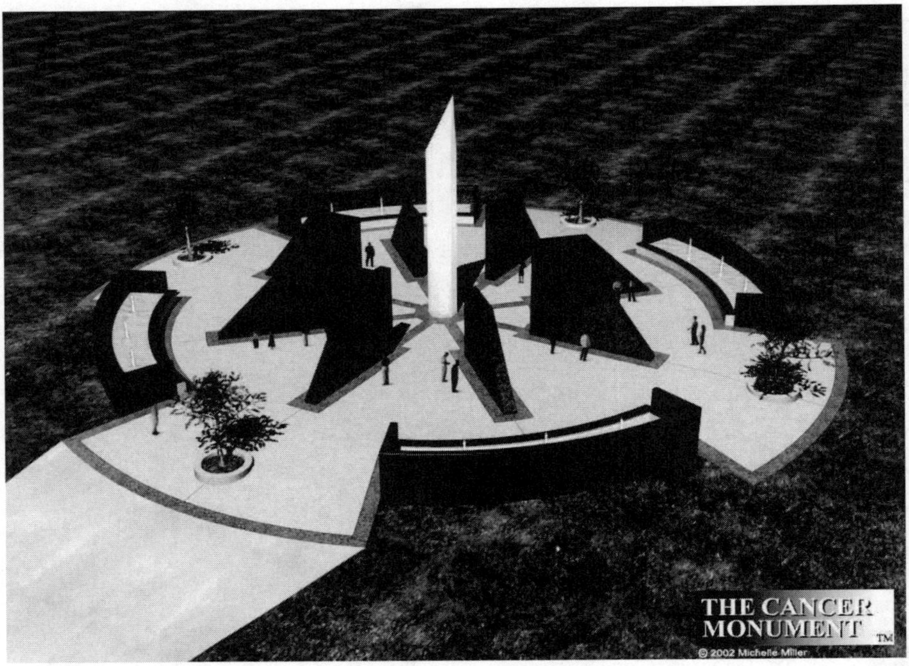

"You must be the change you wish to see in the world."
—Mahatma Gandhi

Chapter 4
Forward March!

One September morning as I drove to work, I contemplated topics for Graduate research papers and mentally rehearsed October meetings with city officials in Allen about the future of The Cancer Monument. The air was crisp that morning as the leaves began their annual show of brilliant orange and yellow. School children skipped along the sidewalks and laughed with their friends on the way to another day of study about the world they'd inherit. I channel-surfed radio stations as I made my way through traffic and happened upon a station that I supposed had run out of fresh ideas for skits.

"Two planes crashed into the World Trade Towers and terrorism is suspected," the announcer said. Horror and confusion was heard in the background as a live announcer on the scene described what happened while sirens and screams filled my car. Then, there was more talk of a hijacked plane that hit the Pentagon. I turned the dial in disgust for what I thought was a cheap, shock-jock prank, an Orson Welles "War of the Worlds" type skit designed to prey upon public fears and gain ratings. I searched for a station with music and heard the same reports on every radio station. I called Joey on my cell phone and he confirmed that it wasn't a hoax. I dialed my mother's work number in New York and she picked up on the first ring. Her voice was controlled but scared. Along with many nurses in the Hudson Valley, my mother was on standby duty with local hospitals in case the city hospitals overflowed with dead and injured. Days later, we learned that two people we knew who'd worked in the towers were missing: Jennifer, a cousin, and Joe, a family friend. Their bodies were never recovered. Just a week earlier, my parents had laughed and danced with Joe at the wedding of a mutual friend. Joe had become a father again in middle age, and as he held his baby, he and my father set a date to ride their motorcycles together when the autumn foliage would be in all its glory.

"I'm getting on a plane to fly to you right now!" I told my mother.

"You can't. All planes are grounded," she said.

"Well, then, I'm driving to New York!"

"No!" she warned, "Stay where you are. We don't know what's going on right now and poisonous fumes are all over the city. We don't know if biologic weapons were used. We could be the next targets."

I couldn't believe what my mother said. It all sounded like a movie script. Then she reminded me of every strategic target that surrounded her. A nuclear reactor was just thirty-five miles north of midtown Manhattan and about thirty miles south of Newburgh where my mother worked and most of the family resided. The nuclear reactor supplied New York City with upwards of twenty percent of its electricity. Stewart International Airport was in Newburgh and other smaller airports dotted the valley. West Point and other military installations were just minutes away along with several bridges, a river system and a highway of aqueducts that sent drinking water to New York City. The state capitol in Albany was only a ninety-minute drive from Newburgh. To an enemy, these targets made the Hudson Valley area a site to exact damages of disastrous and possibly even permanent proportions. Such an attack could immeasurably affect the health and socio-economic status of the immediate area, as well as New York City, and the adjacent states of Connecticut, Pennsylvania, and New Jersey.

Who was the enemy? What was their sinister plan and were they as familiar with the vulnerable landscape as we were? At that moment, I was dizzy with a singular realization. On a ruthless whim, my family in New York could be wiped out at any moment along with millions of other innocent people. As I held the phone in my hand, I felt lost in a canyon of rage and helplessness and thought that at any moment my mother might be dead.

"I love you," I said it as if it were my last chance to ever say it to her.

My mother let out a painful wail. "Oh! I love you too."

For a few seconds we both broke down in a confusion of tears and swallowed pain. Who would commit such heinous acts against others? Why? Why? I couldn't see the enemy. I couldn't save my family. I couldn't attack back. It was a lot like cancer.

"What about Ben and Shaun?" I asked.

"I don't know yet. I hope they call me soon with information, but the military can't strike until we know who is responsible for this," my mother said.

At the time of September 11th, Lieutenant JG Edward Benjamin Miller was an Assistant Operations Officer in the Commander Amphibious Squadron 8 on the USS Bataan Naval ship. My other brother was U.S. Army 1st Lieutenant Shaun P. Miller, who was stationed in Germany and in charge of a chemical weapons unit. Three cousins, also in various branches of the military were stationed in Korea, or in international waters, and in the months to come, one was injured during battle in Afghanistan. Shaun had orders to stay in Germany, but if needed would be deployed to the Middle East at any time. Within two weeks after September 11th, Ben's ship was deployed from the Naval base in Virginia and sent to the Mediterranean. Exactly where he'd end up, we didn't know for sure then, and he couldn't tell us much, except the name of his ship. Ben had email during the seven months at sea and informed us from time to time that he was safe, and that parcels of popcorn, nuts, Twizzlers, Fig Newtons, Ho-Hos, Ring-Dings and junk food of any kind were welcomed and appreciated. He was in good spirits, worked out a lot at the ship's gym, but for security reasons could reveal no more than that.

"Loose lips sink ships. Just keep watching CNN," he'd write, "then you'll know exactly where I am and what I'm doing."

I wouldn't know more until almost two years later when Ben and I met for a weekend in New York City, but even after several trays of sushi and several bottles of sake between us, he revealed little to me about his mission except that he'd been twenty miles off the coast of Pakistan and troops of Marines deployed on and off his ship and into the battlegrounds of Afghanistan.

"If I tell you what happened, I have to kill you," he joked.

In the initial days that followed September 11th, everyone was on high alert and prepared for the worst. Where once I had seen no military presence in Dallas, now there were more and more military vehicles on familiar streets. I wasn't sure if I should feel protected or alarmed by this and wondered about the soldiers and the weaponry contained inside the covered military trucks that sped past me.

Then, one day as I left work and walked through the parking lot to my car, two civilian men in an adjacent lot threw practice knives at a large piece of plywood traced with a human form. I pretended not to notice them as I unlocked my car door and got inside. Their muscles tensed with each mighty throw and their bare skin boiled from the combination of a late day Texas sun and a bloody anger that surged beneath it.

I was thankful to be cancer-free that day and though still fatigued from my year of battling cancer, I thanked God for my health as I turned the ignition and prayed for the less fortunate. Physically, I still felt beat up from the months of chemo and radiation, but was getting strong again and my hormones were making a slow come back too. Life would go on despite the despotic forces of foreign terrorism and cancer.

Life had to go on, I thought as I drove home. People would continue to fall in love, get married, and have babies. There'd still be carefree Sunday barbeques in the back yard with lots of corn on the cob and juicy watermelon, as well as birthday parties with gooey cake, red balloons, and silly cone hats. Every May and June there'd still be graduations to play "Pomp and Circumstance" and every July, a parade down Main Street to make each flag-waving, cotton-candy-eating citizen proud.

For sure, there'd be better days ahead for the economy too and we'd all live past this horrible time. We'd have to heal. There was no time to waste when the enemy surrounded us. We'd have to re-group and find a balance within the chaos in order to survive. The enemy had knocked us to the ropes in a surprise attack, but we were not down for the count, I told myself. We'd make a better plan and would not go easily into the night. Our mission would be based upon the higher ethics of justice and freedom, and with it, we'd destroy the enemy.

As I continued to drive home, I felt a rush of adrenaline in anticipation of more battle ahead and mentally prepared myself for anything. Like a review of basic training, I tried to remember scenes and interviews from war documentary films or books that I'd read for history classes. I tried to remember what the survivors had done, whether a soldier, or civilian. Where did they hide, how did they cope through, and beyond war? They stayed calm. That strategy seemed to be constant. I remembered the advice that my brothers gave to me a year earlier when I was diagnosed with cancer. I told them that my strategy to cope, fight, and survive was to think like a soldier. "I'm a soldier in the War on Cancer," I said.

"That's for damn sure! The only difference is that you can't see your enemy," they'd tell me.

In the months to come, I'd tell them details about my cancer treatments as well as the scientific and technical advances made in the War on Cancer. It was both amazing and foreign to them, but was now a part of my every day. Cancer was my morning reveille and roll call. I told them about mine-sweep missions that I carried out as I searched for hot spots of cancer cells throughout the landscape of my body. I'd tell them about hand-to-hand combat and the most ruthless conversations that one can have with an enemy who desires every ounce of your breath, every cell, and the life force of your beating heart.

Nearly twenty years earlier, Lance Corporal Mike Miller had been a Recon Force Marine. "Once a Marine, always a Marine," he'd say. With talk of military strategy and combat, Mike's language turned to military jargon and in an instant he was a Marine again in the jungles of South America as he talked to me about how to fight a mortal enemy. Mike told me about helicopters that dropped him into the sea with a partially deflated raft, a compass and a handful of men to carry out stealth missions onto foreign shores. In the dark canopy of the Central American jungles, he conducted seven missions in dangerous, forsaken areas of Nicaragua, Guatemala, and El Salvador. He told me about loneliness and isolation mixed with the constant bite of voracious bugs. The bacteria and other fungi spawned like an alien mutation and found the warm wetness of his booted feet to be a perfect host. At night, Mike and his men had only a small canopy for cover and at all times, his gun was cocked to protect him.

I didn't want to know the secret of his military missions. I was interested in a far greater secret. "How did you cope through it?" I asked him. I'd ask Ben and Shaun the same question. Early on, I learned that survival in battle was as much mental as it was physical and a lot like when we played war as kids. Stealth was an absolute requirement in a death match regardless if the target was human, or cancerous. Careful study would reveal the enemies vulnerable points: what they ate, daily habits, natural resources, fighting strategy, and what they cherished most of all. With such information, you could slowly weaken the enemy, or strike to annihilate in a quick ambush that would secure your ultimate victory.

"I wish we had more soldiers like you," my brothers would tell me. "You're relentless!"

"I don't take too kindly to invaders, whether cancer or human," I'd say. "There's only room enough for me in this body."

That September day in 2001 as I drove away from the knife-throwers, I remembered the soldiering advice that each brother gave me during my first year of cancer: Mike reminded me of the Marine's motto;

"Swift, Silent and Deadly."

"That's like cancer itself," I said to him one day.

"Yes, it is. And just like a Marine you'll have to match the enemy's force in order to fight back. You have to be worse than the enemy in order to win. You have to be more blood thirsty, more destructive, and you cannot stop. If the enemy has a chance, they'll kill you. Remember that. Be first. Search and destroy. Kill them before they kill you," Mike said.

In 1998, Ben launched missiles into Iraq from his Navy ship.

"Follow orders and remember your training," he told me. "You've got to forget that you're in a war. You're there to do a job. That's it. Just think of it like that when the shit hits the fan and missiles are flying over your head and your men are dead all around you. Remember all the practice drills and all the manuals that you studied. Remember your sergeant who screamed in your face when you did it wrong. You can't fall apart under fire, or else you're finished."

I not only applied this methodology to my own life, but realized too the importance of public cancer education efforts in the War on Cancer and the role that it played. Cancer prevention and awareness through such things as screenings, lectures, films, and literature is the closest thing we have to a boot camp training ground and yet, it's not enough.

My youngest brother Shaun also gave me important advice, which became an essential part of my early thinking during cancer and an instrumental aspect of The Cancer Monument philosophy, "Duty, Honor and Country. A soldier never forgets the mission and never leaves a fallen comrade."

I was relieved to be cancer-free, but as I drove home that day, I considered the consequences of further attacks on our nation. I considered the possibility of mass hysteria in the streets as tanks rolled past and the enemy surrounded us. How would I move through it and what if I couldn't find Joey in all of the chaos? I imagined people fleeing with possessions strapped to their backs, children in tow and some crying in desperation because they'd been lost in a panicked mob. There'd be many horrors to witness as thousands fled to an ambiguous safety. Our infrastructures, institutions and our entire way of being were all in jeopardy due to the insanity of terrorists with a single desire for total destruction. The scenes I imagined had been the reality of many innocent people in foreign lands, and I hoped that it would never be mine to endure. I was glad to no longer be hooked to an I.V. pole and if necessary, I was ready to defend my life and home in a bloody hand-to-hand combat with this new terrorism. More than anything, I wanted to fly to New York to see my family.

Finally, scheduled flights returned and I arranged to fly to New York at the end of September. I wouldn't see my parents that trip because they flew to Germany to be with Shaun. Mike met me at the airport in Albany and though we wanted to drive to the city to see the wreckage for ourselves, the news cautioned people against it. As we drove to Newburgh we stopped at a diner for lunch and talked non-stop about what had happened on September 11th and what might come.

We remembered how in 1997, we rented a limo and surprised our parents on their wedding anniversary with dinner at Windows on The World Restaurant located on the 107th floor of Tower 1 at the World Trade Center. Joey, Mike's wife, Gloria, my Grandmother Miller and Aunt Joyce joined us. That June evening, the Tower elevator sped us to the 107th floor in seconds. We all let out a 'Whoa!" and braced ourselves. Our stomachs tickled and our eardrums crackled as we soared above the city to what would become for many reasons, an unforgettable memory. Amid impeccable food, wine, the comfort of plush surroundings, and white-gloved service, our spirits soared. That night we laughed at what a bunch of idiots the terrorists were in 1993 to think that they could blow up the World Trade Center tower from the parking garage.

Though my visit to New York was brief, I was relieved to see familiar people and landmarks. The Italian restaurant and the Dairy Queen still stood on the corner of Route 52 in Newburgh across from the car wash. Roadside stands of fresh-picked apples, mulled cider, and pumpkins were in familiar places. College students filled the cafes and hipster joints in New Paltz, and the bronze statue of President McKinley greeted residents and visitors at the crossroads in Walden, as it always had. As my plane lifted into the air on its way back home to Joey and Texas, the landscape was crimson with autumn foliage. My eyes burned with tears as I peered through the plane window like a wondrous child.

"Keep it safe," I prayed. "I want to come back again."

In the weeks that followed 9-11, I was filled with another great concern. With all the financial efforts and charitable monies going to the relief efforts of September 11th, well-established charities suffered from a lack of donations. I'd just formed my Board of Directors for The Cancer Monument and begun the process to become a non-profit organization. Official efforts to fund and build the monument were underway and several meetings in October with the City of Allen, as well as lawyers and other professionals, had been in preparation since the summer.

Now, with recent world events being what they were, a few people offered me kind words of caution: "It isn't a good time to start a new non-profit organization," and "worse economic times are ahead for us all," they predicted.

I didn't listen. The Cancer Monument was the people's monument. If the people wanted The Cancer Monument, then it would be built. The problem was that enough of the public didn't know about it yet. One thing was certain: 60,000 Honoree names wasn't an impossible quest when tens of millions battled cancer worldwide. My role was to make The Cancer Monument possible, but many elements had to come together before Honoree names could be gathered from across the country.

Though I had the vision of the monument locked inside my head, I wasn't a skilled artist. I needed an architect who could help bring my vision into technical drawings so that engineers and other building specialists like granite workers, lighting, and water specialists and others could erect it. Then, there was the matter of land: a place had to be located and a process worked out with local government. Community relations across all business sectors had to begin from scratch, as well as an entire organizational structure developed, budgets made, fundraising efforts, and the development and implementation of a national media and marketing plan.

Lots of volunteers were needed to carry out these roles. That I knew of, such a feat had never been done before by a grass-roots organization. There was no handbook, no model and no one to pick up the phone and mentor me on how to carry out these efforts. In the autumn of 2001, the Foundation had no financial sponsorship, minimal volunteer support and no ability to garner media. We jumped up and down, virtually unnoticed and unknown in a great sea of national public interest groups. We were sustained by our conviction that regardless of world political and economic events, the time had come for The Cancer Monument. The Cancer Monument deserved to be built and the public had a right to know about it.

As if a test of faith, disaster struck again.

<u>October 26, 2001</u>

Happy Halloween, my cancer is back. It seems like a bad joke. I am so tired of this cancer crap.

***

The news that cancer had made a return took us all by surprise. For less than a minute, I lost my composure in Dr. Smith's office and swore like a trucker, a sailor, a pirate, anything but a lady. Cancer was back on the radar screen in only six months. It had never left. I'd worked so hard to win and all of it, the worry, the puking, the two extra months of chemo that I volunteered for meant nothing. In that moment of truth, I felt worthless. Defeated. Helpless. I burst into tears and apologized to Joey for knowing me in the first place. It was a pathetic, though thankfully brief scene, and even Dr. Smith fought back tears.

Joey assured me that he loved me more than ever. "We're a team and together we'll get through it," he said.

That was my rainbow in the storm. I was furious at the entire situation and in that moment, I recommitted myself to battle with the knowledge that Joey was ready to fight with me. Cancer was unfair. Yes, that was true. But there was no time to brood over that obvious point, when raw, fast action was needed. Cancer hadn't gotten the message that I was in charge. It had lived quiet and unnoticed in my body for an unknown length of time, maybe forever. After the initial shock came a stronger emotion: I was ready to kick cancer's ass like never before. I was pissed off for its ability to overtake and hold me hostage. I was pissed off that I'd been emotionally ambushed even for a minute at the news of its return, and vowed that I'd never allow it again. I was willing to play this dirty game one more time and with it, I'd shed every last drop of blood to strike a visceral vengeance against cancer. I was in need of a strategy and a plan.

"So what happens now?" I asked Dr. Smith. "Is there a plan, or are you going to tell me to go home and make funeral arrangements?"

Dr. Smith talked about bone marrow transplants. The only thing I knew about marrow was that wild animals and my dog Buddy, liked to chew on bones to get at it. I didn't understand what bone marrow had to do with my treatment plan, but Joey and I were about to receive a crash course education on yet another area of cancer.

Stem cell transplants were a next step in the attack plan against blood related cancers like Lymphomas when standard chemo and radiation protocols failed. After an hour with Dr. Smith, we were dizzy with new information that came at an urgent pace and in medical jargon unfamiliar to us. There was no time to waste when cancer cells multiplied. Dr. Smith explained that bone marrow transplants weren't his area of expertise, but from what we understood thus far, it sounded like I'd be leveled to a place close to death and then retrieved back to life. We'd learn much more from the experts, which meant that I'd be in the care of a new medical team and a new doctor.

"A new doctor?" I screeched in disbelief and began to cry. "I don't want a new doctor. I only want you. You're my doctor!" I beseeched Dr. Smith as though his helicopter took off, leaving me broken and muddied on a battlefield while the roar of enemy tanks approached and thundered the earth. I'd lost my general. For a few moments, I felt unworthy and abandoned. Albeit a hard-won feat, I'd placed my life in his hands. I trusted him and grew to rely on his calm, assured voice, even his zany humor. I couldn't imagine soldiering on without him. History proved that I couldn't win a war without a great general like Grant, MacArthur, or Schwartzkopf. I felt vulnerable to attack.

For days, the news of another care team caused me to obsess with horrible thoughts and unhinged my dormant insecurities about the medical profession. As I anticipated the next phase of this tactical maneuver against cancer, I knew what I needed most of all: A commander-in chief. I wanted a doctor who was a great leader, an expert, teammate, and when absolute authority and decisive action were needed, I wanted no slackers. I wanted someone who had great concern for me, who saw past the cancer stamp at the top of my medical chart and saw me, the person instead. I could be difficult. I knew that about myself. I wanted a doctor who was a hell of a lot tougher than me on my worst day. I knew my shortcomings in a crisis. I needed a doctor who wouldn't be worn down by my orations and tangents, who'd listen to me, but give it to me straight up with bottom line facts. Most of all, I wanted someone who'd dogfight for me to Mars and back if necessary. I might have been asking too much out of one human being, but I knew what I needed to make it through the battle.

I started chemotherapy the next day and for the next two months, Dr. Smith remained my doctor as I received intense chemo in preparation for a stem cell transplant. The intensity of this new chemo cocktail was a physical crush, worse than any I'd experienced before. I was familiar with the rest of the routine. A medi-port was reinserted into my chest, my hair fell out in two weeks, I was dizzy, out of breath, bruised, lost my balance a lot, slept more than twelve hours a day, or sometimes not at all. Even with anti-nausea medications, my stomach was on fire; I puked my guts for days and drank bottles of Maalox without relief.

This time, I didn't care about my hair loss. I just wanted to be through with cancer and didn't want to be taken by surprise, either, so I prepared for another round of battle in the best way I knew how. I stocked up on foods I knew I'd be able to easily eat like soups with pull tops, packaged instant oatmeal, prunes to combat constipation from chemo, and yogurt. I washed out wigs, brushed off hats, and remembered that I had to buy new sleeping caps so that I wouldn't lose body heat at night, or have my sensitive bald head rub against the pillow. In fact, I took charge of the hair situation one day when my mother visited from New York. She was aghast to find me in the bathroom, with scissors in hand as I hacked off haphazard chunks of shoulder length hair.

"Oh, no, don't cut it," she said.

I was in mid-cut when she walked in.

"Its just hair," I said, "Besides I don't feel like picking it out of my soup and everywhere else for days. There will be less to vacuum when it falls out."

"Okay, well let me at least make a style." It seemed like an unnecessary step to me, but I figured that it was important to my mother, so I sat as she made a short, pretty hairstyle, which would last for less than two weeks before chemo left me bald.

Hair. Big deal, I thought. Cancer. Now that was something to worry about. This chemo round was incredibly difficult and as the night wore on, Joey, my mother and I wound up at the emergency room because of the pain I experienced. A few hours later, I was home again and twisted and turned on the couch unable to find comfort. For days, I'd been incredibly weakened by chemo, unable to brush my teeth, shower, and hadn't even the strength to change my underwear. A thought crossed my mind: Children.

The next day, Joey wheeled me into the fertility clinic. We arrived with the hope that we might store some eggs before the stem cell transplant, but never imagined the finality of the doctor's answers. The doctor explained that my platelets were too low to risk an egg-harvesting procedure and that I might bleed to death if my blood couldn't coagulate. Also, the insertion of a foreign object into my body increased the risk of bleeding and infection, and both posed deadly risks for a procedure that was not life urgent, according to the doctor. But in my opinion, this was all about the urgency of many unborn lives that would never be if I didn't retrieve some eggs that day. The doctor refused to do the procedure. I would have removed the darn eggs myself if I had a scalpel and enough energy. I urged the doctor one last time and didn't care about bleeding to death all over his office. I was on the verge of no logic when Joey reminded me that I wouldn't be a mother at all if I were dead.

The doctor explained that because my hormone levels hadn't made a complete return before I was hit again with more chemo, it was unlikely that a menstrual cycle would ever return after the bone marrow transplant. Even if my eggs were remotely viable, they'd be further compromised once thawed years later for fertilization.

"There's a 99% chance of irreversible ovarian failure as a result of the bone marrow transplant," the doctor said.

"But, we never had a chance to have a baby," I said, as if that point made any difference at all to the more serious situation at hand - cancer.

Joey and the doctor talked about all kinds of other parenting options for us to explore. I stopped listening, but I heard the word adoption through tears that stung like embedded shrapnel, and I saw Joey smile. From the moment of my cancer diagnosis, our dreams to make a family in the old-fashioned way were kidnapped with no ransom note. From the beginning, we asked questions and followed medical advice, but fate had a different plan for us. Infertility would be the unfortunate price to pay for a cancer-free life.

***

Society and religion teaches that a woman's value in the world centers around her ability to marry and produce children. With every stage of cancer, I stepped back to review and question my feminine worth against the norm and as a result of infertility, even more so. Believe it or not, I still struggled with some old, mixed-up ideas, and though it wasn't the first time I heard my husband's more open-minded point of view on these matters, I was still incredulous over the fact that I was valuable to Joey merely because I existed. It didn't matter to him whether I had hair, or no hair, extra pounds, chipped nail polish, matching shoes and purse, or was infertile. In Joey's opinion, the fact that my heart still beat was cause enough to celebrate, but I continued to throw my anchor among the rocks of old ideologies. In doing so, I remained tangled in a deflated definition of womanhood and was unable to sail with the current of the new normal. Infertility exacerbated my philosophical confusions because since I was a little girl, I envisioned myself as a mother in one way - the old fashioned way.

Yet again, I had to readjust my self-concept because of cancer. Over the next couple of years, I asked myself many questions on the topic of motherhood. Did I still want to be a mother and if so, how would the new normal align with parenthood? Joey, on the other hand, didn't doubt my ability and was entirely more flexible with a definition of himself as husband and father, which made it easier for him to look to the future and move past the loss. The bottom line, he reminded me, was that he loved me no matter what, and that my health was a priority more important than any feminine ideals, or the cultural norms that I still clung to. "Our wedding vows said nothing about children. It's about you and me," Joey reminded one day. "I'm not married to your ovaries and I can't have a marriage by myself, so let's get you healthy and think about a family later."

Life sounded so easy when said like that. Within the safety of my marriage, I felt like a desirable and complete woman. Still, from time to time, I couldn't help but remember our first date when we talked about marriage and children while seated at a restaurant table over steak and shrimp. Joey captured my heart that evening when he welled with tears to describe how he planned to teach his son to play basketball. For his daughter, he'd show through the years that she was the most precious little girl who'd never feel inferior in the world, or be mistreated by any man because she had the love of the best man of all - her daddy. With that, I knew that I'd found my prince.

Infertility was a part of my new normal, and later I'd learn that I wasn't alone. Since 1997 over ten million Americans who've battled cancer are alive and many of those people are now faced with infertility as a result of their cancer treatments. Repeatedly, patients say that they were never told of the prospect of infertility until it was too late to take precautionary measures. In a 2003 journal report relating to the preservation of fertility in young cancer patients, Philip M. Rosoff, M.D., and Melanie L. Katsur, J.D., from Duke University state that while more than 70% of children and young adults are cured of their cancers, infertility is commonly the most long-term, damaging effect to quality of life. Medical professionals have a medical, legal and ethical responsibility to help prevent this side effect for patients, survivors, and families. Infertility will continue to be an issue for cancer survivors so long as chemotherapy and other harsh procedures are the standard treatment protocol. Treating the whole patient should include a concern for all areas of their lives that may be impacted by cancer. Patient education should include a discussion about family planning and if at all possible, preventive measures taken to store eggs or sperm before cancer therapies begin.

Though the doctors held a fragmentary hope that nature might make a comeback for me, they explained the medical improbability. True, there were cases of healthy, beautiful babies born to post-cancer couples that had once been told that they were infertile, but with regard to bone marrow transplants, that hope would be exceptionally remote. Joey and I wouldn't waste time on false, miniscule hopes, or subscribe to the fairy tale club of wishes made upon a shooting star, or those made somewhere over the rainbow. In this matter like others, we lived in the honest world of facts in order to move forward and make new realities. If God produced a miracle, we'd be grateful for it. In the meantime, we weren't about to have the undertow of infertility drag us out to sea. So for the time being, we moved beyond that crisis to deal with the more urgent one at hand. In less than a month, I'd have a bone marrow transplant. As January 2002 ticked closer, we celebrated the holidays, attended New Year's Eve parties with friends and happily said goodbye to 2001.

***

A new medical care team meant new relationships, more trust, and new lines of communication about even the most trivial, embarrassing, and personal matters. As Dr. Agura entered the examination room and reached out his hand to shake mine for the first time, I mechanically obliged, though hesitant. My heart pounded with old fears and cynicism for any doctor's ability to cure me. In the days prior, Joey and I spent time working through my emotional issues, the fact that there was only so much that we could control, and the rest we'd trust to God and the doctors. At the beginning of my cancer journey, trust was a weak area for me and was no different more than a year and a half later with my life on the line again. I knew that I couldn't battle cancer alone, but I didn't want a new doctor. I didn't want to place my life in the hands of strangers, but my urgent situation required it.

Before my bone marrow transplant, I never considered how blood was made. It was just there. "Bone marrow is an organ that's found in the cavities of bones. It resembles blood and contains stem cells, which produce red cells, white cells, and other blood components," Dr. Agura said. He explained a great many things to Joey and me in understandable terms and even drew pictures when needed. I liked that he drew pictures. With the doctor's confidence presiding over the room, I felt my shoulders decompress from somewhere up around my ears. Though only pencil drawings, the visual was enough to understand the concept behind the bone marrow transplant. I had walked into the initial consultation with Dr. Agura with a negative attitude and no confidence, but now my fears were gone. I was excited to have a new general in the War on Cancer and was ready to march forward, armed with an aggressive, but riskier plan of attack.

Peripheral blood stem cells were to be harvested from my own bone marrow before the transplant, then frozen, stored, and returned to my body after all existing marrow had been destroyed by two weeks of high-dose chemo. I'd be brought down to a level close to death, but blood transfusions and antibiotics would swoop in to rescue me. The idea was that hi-dose chemo would kill all existing cancer cells and the peripheral, or seedling blood cells that were frozen and stored would be re-entered into my body to embed, sprout, and grow new healthy, cancer-free blood. This process of growing new blood would take weeks. There were no guarantees either.

A battery of cardio-pulmonary and other tests were conducted to see if I could physically endure the procedure. The doctor explained that I'd be very sick, much sicker than before, but would feel progressively better as the months went by and make a full recovery in about a year. I couldn't fathom being that sick. Unlike a donor bone marrow transplant, the risk of death was minimal for an Autologous transplant and because I was young, strong, and feisty, I was told that I'd probably do well during the transplant and recover. I was skeptical about the fifty percent success rate though,

"Flip a coin," I said to Dr. Agura, "those are my odds of success." At the outset of my cancer battle I stood confident with an overwhelming 90% chance of success. Now, I felt outnumbered by the mediocre odds of a stem cell transplant.

"Well, if you can't be optimistic, then, I'll be optimistic for you," the doctor said.

I got my wish. I had a doctor that would fight for me when I couldn't fight for myself and one who'd dish it back to me as well as I could dish it out. With no other treatment options available to me, I took my chances and hoped to say goodbye to cancer forever.

The ordeal of a stem cell transplant made my first year of chemo and radiation look like a pony ride at the county fair. We stayed in a hospital-owned, fully furnished apartment around the corner from the hospital and my mother stayed with us for two weeks. Every day, the three of us went to the cancer center for the transplant. For over a month, Joey went back and forth between the cancer center, his job, and home for clean clothes, not to mention grocery trips and late-night pharmacy runs and back downtown again to the hospital. Our friends Rebecca and Paul watched our dog, Buddy, during that time and we were so grateful to know that our beloved pet was in safe, loving hands as we endured more crisis.

The fact that I had cancer made my mother want to do everything for me at first.

"Just because I have cancer doesn't mean I'm helpless," I'd say. Though it took me much longer to do ordinary things while on chemo, I preferred to be self-sufficient.

"Well, let me do something for you," she'd plead. We'd go back and forth about whether I needed help fixing a meal, or getting dressed, or getting in and out of a car, or whether I wanted Joey to bring the dreaded shower bench from home. Did I want to walk down the long hallways of the hospital to the bone marrow clinic, or did I want a wheelchair instead?

"I can do it myself," I snipped one day in frustration as my mother poured me a glass of juice. Joey and I had developed a synchronized dance of sorts with each other and our medical team; my mother struggled to find the best way to help out. In the day-to-day of a constant cancer crisis, Joey knew my limitations, knew that I was independent and preferred it that way. He knew that help from others wouldn't be taken at all unless it was sincere and offered with loyal intent. I wouldn't be anyone's charity case. I had pride, dignity, and self-worth. Most of all, I needed to be the leader of my own life. At worst, I needed the illusion of a choice if none were possible.

But, there were a few times when I no longer had either. In those instances, my ego stepped in to defend its territory and I needed to be reminded of who was in charge of the stem cell transplant. One day, I was in dire need of a two units of blood. I refused to have the transfusion. I protested and debated my reasons against it with nurses and even with Dr. Agura at my bedside until he explained the consequences to me: organ failure and brain damage could result without a blood transfusion. With that, there was no longer any debate. I tempted the rules on another occasion when, with my hand on my hip and hooked to an I.V., I hotly protested to Laura Brougher, Dr. Agura's nurse, that if required, 'I simply would not have full body radiation treatment.' She educated me as to why the procedure was used as I continued to bargain like a tourist at a Turkish bazaar. Then, she delivered the bottom line: "If Dr. Agura feels that you need it for a successful transplant, then there will be no negotiation," she finished. Whomp! I wasn't in charge. As it turned out, I didn't need the radiation after all, but I learned a lesson in hospital democracy that day. As a patient, I had choices. However, in certain cases, there was no room for two generals. The doctor was in charge and democracy was suspended. There'd be no lobbying, no bargaining, or new policy-making, except for one; my illness took precedence over the demands of ego. I didn't have to be in charge of this one. My doctor had me covered. I had to follow orders and trust his leadership. I was in safe, capable hands, and now I knew it. I felt a mountain of worry lift.

As chemotherapy knocked me down to abysmal levels, my mother's stress level rode new heights. Every day when the lab reports came, her eyes widened and she grew pale at the reality on paper.

"Oh, my God, they're killing her," my mother would say to Joey in alarm. My blood counts dropped closer and closer to zero. This was normal for the procedure. Dr. Agura, Laura Brougher, and others on the Bone Marrow Team were always a calm presence. When we were nervous, they'd remind us of the steps in the process and assured us that the plummet of red and white blood cells were necessary in order to destroy the existing marrow and bring it to ground zero. Then, healthy stem cells could be reintroduced back into the body to grow new, and we hoped, cancer-free blood.

For a person who'd had nothing more than a tonsillectomy and a root canal, the bone marrow transplant was the most extreme physical assault I'd ever had. I took notice of the fact that a crash cart rested in the center of the nurses' station, though I figured that it was there for the other patients, some of whom were visibly much worse off than me.

Every day, Laura Brougher and one of the doctors came to talk to us. They reassured us that my transplant was on target. In those moments of emotional crisis, when mere common sense and especially new information was difficult to remember, the Baylor Bone Marrow Team repeated information as many times as we needed. We asked a lot questions. Some were off-the-wall crazy, others were rooted in fear or ignorance, and all were answered with as much weight as those questions that were more obviously intelligent. When the doctors weren't around, Laura seemed to be at the receiving end of most of our questions. She was fabulous at teaching and helping us understand. After a while, we prefaced every question with an apology, "Gee, I know that I've already asked you this question fifteen times, but…"

The Bone Marrow Team encouraged us to re-read the thick patient information manual we'd been given about bone marrow transplants and they continued to instruct and guide us with a variety of visual diagrams, including a calendar marked off to count the days until I'd receive my own stem cells back. The nurses were a constant bright light in our day and helped to make our collective worst nightmares a more tolerable situation.

Sharon, a nurse's aide, kept us smiling every day with funny stories and had many pairs of interesting shoes, which created conversations about fashion, shopping and gratefully, not cancer. I'm not sure that Sharon ever knew how important this was for me, but she did know that I preferred the private room as opposed to the curtained rooms and she fluffed up my pillow every morning at the bone marrow clinic. I was glad to be cared for and treated with dignity and respect. All resources and methods of support were available to us at Baylor, including nutritionists and social workers and whenever any questions arose, they'd research it and come back with a wealth of information.

For over twenty-five years, my mother had been a nurse and her stressed exhales were a constant reminder that I was in a dangerous situation. She read the patient information manuals over and over, talked to my doctors and soon became as informed as Joey and I were about bone marrow transplants. My mother soon found her niche. Before my transplant began, Dr. Agura asked me if I'd participate in a clinical trial. I wanted to do my part for research but was reluctant at first until it was explained that the trial was to test for a new drug that prevented sores in the mouth and digestive tract, a common problem for many cancer patients. Aside from being incredibly painful, this type of sore could prevent a patient from receiving proper nutrition in a critical time. It was my mother's job to administer the drug and record the information for the two-week study. We felt very proud to be involved in a clinical trial and hoped that one day, our small role might assist the process of FDA approval and maybe save lives.

Every day, the researcher came to deliver the vials that I was to swish and swallow every two hours. After several days, we presumed that I received the drug instead of a placebo because I had no mouth sores. One day, my mother, the doctor, and a researcher beamed as I chomped away at a chicken sandwich. I gave them all a quizzical look as they crowded the small room with smiles and remarked upon how hearty my appetite was during the transplant. I felt silly about it but later realized how important this really was. My appetite had been exceptional throughout my illness and as a result I gained weight, especially since I had been unable to exercise. Though the extra weight depressed me, my doctors were pleased about it and scolded me when I threatened to crash diet.

"Cancer isn't a weight loss program," the doctors reminded me. "This is no time to be on a diet."

They'd describe how lucky I was to have extra fat since many cancer patients had lost half their body weight and were fed through tubes. As a result, some were too weak to receive, or endure the hardship of a life-saving bone marrow transplant, and died. Nutrition is a serious matter during cancer and though I felt like a two-year-old when they applauded my victory over a chicken sandwich, it was an important way to measure progress. I took responsibility for this area of my health, as I always had, and journaled my food, vitamin, supplements, and water intake throughout the transplant and tracked calories, fat, protein, calcium and other nutrients. The medical staff appreciated this because it helped them, but though my appetite was good and my mental alertness high, physically, I felt dead.

The fact that my heart beat at all was a daily wonder to me. The level of hardship placed on my body was incredible and beyond what I had ever imagined. I had no energy and mentally dragged myself through every fragmented step of every day during the transplant: bite, chew, swallow, breathe, turn the channel, put one foot in front of the other, sit up, stand up, breathe again. Every spoken sentence required forced energy. I'd drag my I.V. cart behind me to the bathroom and back to bed encouraging myself with lots of self-talk with each step: You can do it. You're strong. You'll make it. If nothing else, just keep thinking, I'd repeat inside my head. Though I felt like a carcass, I still took time to enjoy the beauty of a new fallen snow one February day as it blanketed Dallas in a display of large chunks of fluffiness. As I trod from the car into the apartment after hours of treatment at the bone marrow clinic, snow hit my face and in the moment of that icy splash, I was reminded that I was alive and was grateful.

"Well, I never thought that I'd see snow it Texas," my mother said.

"Enjoy it while it lasts, it'll be gone by tomorrow," I said.

Then, more disastrous news hit. A friend and co-worker of Joey's named Chet was hospitalized on a different floor and hung close to death. Chet was in his late thirties and was a heavy smoker. He suffered a stroke one evening and hours after his admittance to the hospital he slipped into a vegetative state and was put on life-support. Joey kept a close eye on Chet before his family from Louisiana made it to Dallas. Chet was unconscious, bloated beyond recognition, and tubes and wires seem to obliterate the fact that a human being existed. In a single moment, his life had changed forever. Returning to the Bone Marrow unit from Chet's hospital room, Joey looked frightened and overwhelmed. His eyes glazed and he was so pale that I thought he'd collapse.

"Why don't you get out of this hospital, take a drive, and sleep at home tonight. Look at all the doctors and nurses around me. I'll be fine," I said. Joey nodded blankly. He was in need of escape, if only for a night. Chet's prognosis became much worse and his family had to make the unfortunate decision to take him off life support. He died a week later.

***

With a compromised immune system from high-dose chemo, I had no ability to fight off infections during my transplant. For weeks, I was forced to wear a surgical mask to protect myself from others. Germ warfare during a stem cell transplant meant constant hand washing, no fresh flowers, or plants, and all fresh fruits and vegetables had to be washed before they entered my living space. Visitors, especially children, were not encouraged because of the great infection risk they posed to me and other patients.

With my mother around, germs didn't stand a chance. Our apartment was practically a sterile environment. At the cancer center, my mother continued her patrol for the possibility of any infractions and unsanitary conditions that might come in contact with me. After a week, she loosened her grip a bit and admitted that the bone marrow transplant team at Baylor was an exceptional group and superior to the emergency room staff we'd experienced at a North Dallas hospital.

There, she had spotted improper nursing procedures and let it be known, "That's the third mistake I've seen you make in under an hour. You want to try it again?" Jet-lagged and stressed my mother was in no mood to be polite at 2:00 a.m. "You uncapped that needle too soon. You might as well throw it out now that the tip has touched the counter. Do you know how many germs are on the surface of that counter? That's how easily deadly Staph is transmitted!" she scolded. With decades of nursing and teaching behind her, my mother was on the lookout for mistakes. She found none at the Baylor bone marrow unit during her stay and remarked to everyone back in New York that I was very fortunate to live in Dallas where such great medical care was available and only a short distance from where I lived.

During my transplant, what I saw reflected back in the mirror was a stranger. The far-away look in my eyes frightened me most of all. Except for the fact that my personality was strong, my body felt like a fragment that might extinguish from this plane of existence at any moment. It would be several months before a sparkle returned to my face. In the meantime, my skin color was a ghastly white and every physical effort was as though the weight of twenty elephants was upon me. Every morning when I woke up, I was surprised to still be alive. From the balcony of the Dallas apartment I took inventory of the bustle and noise of life around me in order to be reassured that I was really here. Though the future of each week was a mystery, I was happy to be alive.

As the transplant procedure wore on, I became more conscious of the fact that death was a possibility and had to reconcile myself to it. I wasn't ready to die. I'd tell myself and God that I had two feet firmly planted on this earth and wasn't interested in that kind of journey for a long while. Eighty-eight, now that's a good age to die, I'd think. I could do a lot between now and then.

I wanted to go home to my own bed and the taste of water from my own glasses. I wanted to be next to the protective calm of my dog, Buddy, who I was sure had forgotten me. I'd call my friend, Rebecca, just to hear a voice from the outside world and so that Buddy could hear my voice too and know that I was okay. Afterwards, I'd hang up the phone, cry and felt like a bad dog mother.

The sicker I got, the more determined I became to get healthy again, and always, thoughts of The Cancer Monument fueled my march forward. I did not fear cancer. I despised it and hoped that the high-dose chemo I took would choke the life out of it once and for all. Cancer didn't obey rules. It had no respect for life. In the absence of rules and with no court to convict me, I could be as rebellious as I wanted in a deadly game with a faceless stranger.

In the months ahead, I'd often remember the wise words of a couple of World War II veterans who sat on opposite sides of me one afternoon in Dr. Smith's office as we all had our chemo cocktails. Though in their golden years, the physical stature of these men was nothing short of Texas-sized and there was evidence enough that they'd once been a tremendous presence on a battlefield. That day, I struggled through a rare pity party, had already gone through a box of tissues, and gave my apologies to the two men for hot, angry tears that wouldn't stop, no matter how hard I tried.

"Aw, go ahead and cry honey," said one man as he put his hand on mine to console me. "I've cried a lot of tears myself over this. This cancer is worse than any enemy I ever shot with a gun. At least then I could see my enemy coming and stood a chance. With cancer, it's an inside fight and a much tougher enemy than I ever imagined."

The other veteran nodded in agreement and said, "This is a different kind of fight and it takes every aspect of your being to win. You can do it," he encouraged. "Just aim at your target, shoot, and keep marching forward."

My tears went away to be next to such heroic men, and as chemo dripped through my veins, I was in awe to hear their stories of brave battle in Europe. Though we were decades apart in age, we now fought the same enemy and together we were soldiers. They filled me with inspiration and I left the cancer center that day feeling proud. I never saw them again and whenever I asked about them no one knew who they were. Whoever those men were, I've called them "my angels" ever since. I'd always be ready for battle and through the legacy of The Cancer Monument others would be renewed with hope, courage, and inspiration too.

From my laptop and sick bed, I continued to organize the Foundation. I planned for a variety of meetings in the months ahead, including one with an architect whom I'd located months earlier. The fact that I needed an architect at all was a point that filled me with concern and for over a year. I delayed the matter. I was deadlocked on this single issue: I wanted to protect the purity of the monument and would not consent to latitudes with its design. I was worried that an architect might attempt to do so. Regardless of my inhibitions, The Cancer Monument needed to exist and needed to leave the protection of my mind.

I now understood how mothers feel when their child steps onto a school bus for the first time. In that moment of separation, pride, and truth, you realize that your child is now fully in the world. So, in November 2001, I made a series of calls from a long list of Dallas architects. Only one man called me back. Only one man was supposed to, Danny McLarty. A spiritual man, Danny felt that God played a big part in his survival from prostate cancer and for that he was grateful for a renewed life. From the moment I first talked to Danny about The Cancer Monument, we shared a connection that is difficult to explain. Because I was weakened from chemo, I was not able to meet Danny in person for many months, but we communicated by telephone about the design details and that momentous day in my living room when it was first given to me. To this day, I am in awe about how in sync Danny was with the vision that I explained. I realize, too, as Danny does, that a higher power brought us together for the sake of The Cancer Monument.

***

I am a soldier. I'm alone on a country back road in search of my enemy. My gun is at the ready. On either side of me are miles of cornfields and ahead, only sky. A hawk soars overhead as if to signal the approach of danger. I hear the rumble of many feet and smell the scent of battle. As I come to the top of the road, the scene is clearer. I do not fight alone. Before me is a vast open field prepared for war. On one side is the cancer enemy and on the other, the afflicted. In between is the green earth, which will soon turn to bloody red. I take my position among the other soldiers who will rage upon this enemy of mankind. Some are missing limbs and some have dark circles underneath their eyes from years of stress and worry. Some have only homemade weapons, others have only their bare hands, but we are all there for the same thing - to destroy cancer.

We are soldiers in the War on Cancer. We are there to fight for past wrongs, for disrupted peace, and ravaged innocence. We are there to fight for our present and our future. We are there to fight for our littlest soldiers, too young to be on this battlefield and for the old, too weakened by chemo to bear arms. We will give no mercy to cancer when justice is at stake. There are many millions alongside me now, gathering, gathering, behind and in front of me still more gather. We know that the enemy waits for us just over that hill. The air is heavy and hot with angry tempers. Our weapons are drawn. The sound of our anticipation as we wait for the signal to charge is a deafening roar as many foreign tongues exchange familiar stories of what cancer did to them. With each story, still more gather from the sides of this banded coalition: the caregivers, families, doctors, politicians, clergy, nurses, researchers, and friends. They have all come to fight alongside the diagnosed and the cured. Unless we win this battle, there will be no tomorrow.

I struggle to the front lines to be among the first to strike. My body is tight, my jaw locks, and every muscle prepares for a death match. I do not fear the enemy. I've fought them before. I am not afraid of Death either for we have talked, hand in hand as friends, only to learn that it is not yet my time to die. I am here to fight. Just for now I have suspended reason in order to enter into this killing zone. I wait for the horn to blow. Suddenly, a cool breeze from the north fills my lungs with oxygen as battle commands are yelled from behind me and across the battalions... Soldiers at the ready! Weapons pointed forward! On my command! We are seconds away from battle.

There is much last-minute prayer and rebel yelling among us now as we wait for the final order to charge. My fellow soldiers shout out: Victory! Be gone to hell with you, cancer! But, I have no words. I am long past words. This war is for a good cause, I remind myself. Watch your back and do what you've got to do. Remember your training. My eyes glaze, hands tremble and my mouth waters to pull the trigger and plunge my sword deep, deep, deeper into the bowels of cancer. Oh, how I long to hear them gasp, plead, and moan in agony as we have for so long.

"What are you thinking about?" my mother asked as she glanced up from her book.

"Sushi," I said. "I'm imagining that I'm somewhere else."

***

I wanted more out of life than a private room at a hospital. For weeks during the bone marrow transplant, I thought about what else I'd do when I was well enough to venture out into the world with elevated blood levels and no need to wear a surgical mask. I looked forward to the energy to hold myself upright, to play catch with my dog, and to walk a flight of stairs without exhaustion and the roar of my heartbeat in my ears. As a nurse swabbed and re-dressed the bandages around the medi-port in my chest, I continued to imagine all the goodness of a life that I only hoped was for me. Yet, for some strange reason, I sensed that the battle was not over.

"Joey, I don't think this is over. This transplant isn't going to work," I said.

"What makes you say that?" he asked in astonishment.

"I sense it," I said.

The nurse continued to swab my port and reminded me that attitude was everything. Together, she and Joey were like two cheerleaders in my room.

"What I'm talking about has nothing to do with good versus bad attitude," I told them. "I'm just saying that I think it'll take much more than this to cure me."

Dr. Agura heard about what I said. Later, at my bedside, he told me how important it was for me to stay positive for the battle. "I'm going to be positive for you," he said as he grabbed my socked foot and gave it a playful wiggle.

I understood his point, but I couldn't avoid my intuition. "Sometimes," I said, "a person just knows things."

***

Even though I thought there'd be more battles ahead for me, I hoped that I was wrong. I continued to plan my life, with or without cancer. I wanted to spend more time with Joey. We wanted a spectacular garden with all kinds of herbs and flowers to bloom in every season. Roses. Yes. More roses: red, white, pink, yellow and even orange. The dirt on my hands that day would be my proud reward, I thought. I wanted to take long walks in the park, and as always, Buddy would run ahead with his head held high and his tail wagging.

I wanted to finally see a swimming pool in my back yard, with a waterfall, slide, and floating candles at night. The scent of jasmine would fill the air. We'd have lots of parties, too, like we'd always talked about. Joey wanted costume parties, and zany themes like a "crazy hat" party, or maybe an exotic cultural theme, or a wine tasting. There'd be lots of laughter as we'd all play silly games and the winner and loser would receive corny prizes.

I wanted to have my slender figure back and a skip in my step too. A magnetic allure would make a comeback to each and every cell in my body. I'd look dynamic in a little black dress, heels, sexy red lipstick and my hair up for an evening with Joey, as we'd ride in a beautiful, black limousine through the city. We'd toast my health, smooch, and giggle about our new beginning. I wanted to go to Vegas. I'd never been to Vegas and even though I wasn't a gambler, I still wanted to experience the glitz and glamour of the infamous sin city.

I wanted to travel through Italy, see the Roman ruins, and take a gondola ride in Venice. I wanted to walk through the streets of Jerusalem, tour the Egyptian pyramids of Giza, smell the green of Ireland, feel the fog of England, eat real paella in Spain, taste the coconuts in the South Pacific Islands, and see the Galapagos Islands where Darwin wrote his evolutionary theories.

A horse-drawn carriage ride? Yes. How about that? I had lived in New York for over thirty years and had never taken a carriage ride through Central Park. That would be my reward. Joey and I still hadn't been to Jamaica. I wanted to rest in a hammock and lazily dangle one foot over to squish my toes in the warm sand as the island breeze rocked me. Until I could do all of those things, my imagination was the source of my strength during the weeks of my transplant and the months of recovery afterward. Beyond the beeping sounds of my I.V. cart, a lifetime waited for me outside of the cancer center.

I wanted to finish my Masters degree and maybe, just maybe, even go further to complete a Ph.D. Now that would be something! I wanted to publish, teach, and to help people with cancer to know that through the legacy of The Cancer Monument, an honorable purpose lay within the entangled burden of their diagnosis and that they were heroes of hope, courage and inspiration.

There was one more thing that Joey and I looked forward to - a family of our own. With millions of orphaned children in the world, foreign adoption was an area that we'd continue to explore in the years ahead. We hoped that when the time was right, destiny and circumstance would cross paths and unite us with the child that fate intended to be our own. I imagined the momentous day when our child would be placed in our arms and then, we'd look at each other and no words would be needed.

Though I was bloated from steroids, bald, and a scary shade of white during the stem cell transplant, Joey told me every day that I was beautiful and how much he loved me. My mother, on the other hand, had a hard time with the reality in front of her and whipped out a series of pre-cancer photos to show Dr. Agura and anyone who cared, what her daughter really looked like. I glanced, with little interest to see the remnant of my former self: bright eyes, a carefree smile, full hair, a curvaceous figure, little wisdom, and absolutely no idea of what lay ahead.

My mother seemed to grieve in disbelief as she looked through the pictures. She showed baby pictures and my high school graduation picture too. I didn't want to go down memory lane with her. I had already been through all of that on my own a year earlier and was not going back to a forgotten battlefield, which served me no purpose in my current state of trauma. I was going forward to make new memories and those strong enough to join me in that march were welcomed. But, my mother needed to get through her shock in her own way, at her own pace, and conducted her tour of memory lane with Dr. Agura. She recounted how I'd done this or that as a child, what a good student, and musician I was and all such other bragging rights that mothers feel they have. I sat captive and rolled my eyes with embarrassment.

"Ma! Dr. Agura doesn't want to hear all that. I'll be fine. This is only temporary."

"I just can't believe it," she'd shake her head in disbelief. "Look," she'd say and pointed to a picture as though it offered proof of some kind of alternate reality.

"This one was taken when you were engaged in 1998. This one was taken on your wedding day. You looked so perfect."

"Yeah, and I had cancer, too," I reminded. "In fact, see that picture taken in 1990? I probably had cancer then. And that graduation picture from 1984, I probably had cancer then too," I pointed.

The doctor nodded in agreement and explained that most cancers can take years to grow before symptoms are ever displayed. But now two years after my initial diagnosis, my mother still wanted to know why I had cancer. I had stopped asking that question and was occupied with how to live through it. What caused the one bad cell to misfire and regenerate into millions when no one else in the family had cancer?

Dr. Agura explained that there are several hypotheses, but the exact reasons for cancer are still uncertain. He explained how oncology has come a long way in twenty years because of research, but is far from the answers needed for a cure. The fact that we never saw or heard the impending whirl of a cancer bomb is an illogical point that to this day, Joey, my family, and I still can't comprehend. It was as if one day I was perfectly fine and the next, taken by the ankles and shaken with the force of a rabid cancer beast and then further beaten, gouged, and poisoned daily by cancer therapies in order to be rid of it. How can our culture find protection from cancer? Victory in this war comes in the form of many weapons that work together: Education, prevention, awareness, early diagnosis, psychosocial skills that enable quality of life, and research. Each offers the power of protection and the knowledge needed to thwart the march of a cancerous army.

By the end of February, I was back at home to recover and a month afterward I had strength enough to make social calls again. I was very weak and couldn't leave the house yet. One day, I called a friend and like many people during that time, I hadn't talked to her since January. As I dialed my friend's phone number, I felt a great sense of reward to be back in the stream of life again. At the sound of my voice, hers was distant and cool and her uninterested tone sent a chill through my veins. With every ounce of energy, I'd fought to stay in the world and in that moment, I felt that I was not wanted in it. She didn't want to talk to me and the conversation was over before it began. I wasn't sure what had happened to our friendship in my absence and to this day, I still don't know. A few years earlier, I would have spent a great deal of time, wasted energy, needless guilt, and self-blame in an attempt to mend a soured relationship. But now, whatever the issue was with my former friend, I didn't have the luxury of energy to make her insecurities mine. I had a much greater mystery to uncover. Would my bone marrow transplant work and if it didn't, would I live to see next year?

<u>April 29, 2002</u>

Bad news. My doctor thinks that the cancer has returned based on the latest P.E.T. scan and that I'll need a donor bone marrow transplant. There's a 25% chance that I have a sibling match. I couldn't even cry at the doctor's news. I'm willing to do whatever is necessary just to move on to a new topic in my life. Cancer sucks.

"What if this doesn't work?" was a question that Joey, my mother, and I had asked the doctors in the months before my stem cell transplant. Another bone marrow transplant was the answer except that this transplant would use donor marrow as opposed to my own.

During my transplant months earlier, Dr. Agura advised us all: "Now would be a good time to start talking to all of your relatives about the possibility of being tested as a bone marrow donor. If your cancer comes back, it will come back stronger and there will be no time to waste. If a donor is located both parties would have to drop everything in order to proceed with the transplant." Dr. Agura reminded us how unpredictable cancer cells can be.

"What if a donor can't be found?" we asked.

"We'll cross that bridge when we come to it," said Dr. Agura. Only a few months after that conversation, we crossed the bridge into another unknown battlefield.

My cancer was back. It was unbelievable that it could endure all of that chemo. Now, in the process of a search for a bone marrow donor, the awareness of everyone around me was increased about marrow registries, marrow banks, and how to be a donor. We'd soon share this life-saving message with thousands of people across the country as several bone marrow drives were organized on my behalf.

Bone marrow matches are based on DNA, not blood type. Bone marrow donation is an organ donation whereas blood donation is not. With a simple prick of the finger a donor can be tested. If matched to the recipient, the donor gives life-saving marrow, which soon regenerates; all with no hardship to the donor except for a needle stick and a bruised rear-end. For the recipient, the chance for a new immune system that is able to recognize and destroy cancer cells brings renewed life.

For a successful bone marrow transplant, HLA antigens are needed for a successful match between donor and recipient. This vital fact further complicates the matter because it limits donors to the recipient's ethnic group. The odds of someone finding a perfect match are a million to one. The first likely place to search for bone marrow donors is among full biologic siblings. With each sibling, the odds of a donor match are increased to 25% because of the similar DNA shared between them. That's a heck of a lot better than the lottery! But, when those odds fail, the other place to search for bone marrow donors is through international bone marrow registries. I had no sibling matches.

If. If. If. If. If.

My life had become a series of mathematical probabilities on paper. Hope was the only thing left.

***

SURFACE WARFARE OFFICERS SCHOOL

Newport, Rhode Island

Marrow Program

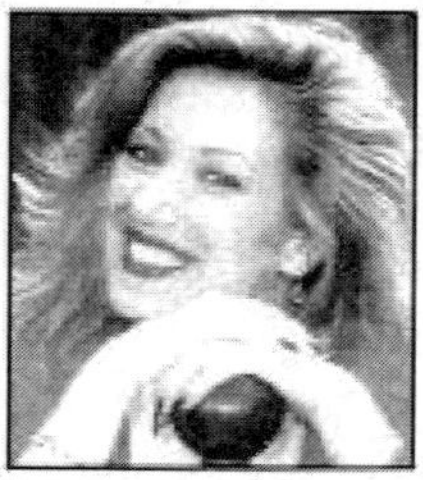

Michelle needs your help!!

Marrow Program

MARROW DONOR REGISTRATION DRIVE

GYM 109

Thursday, 07 November 2002

0900 - 1500

FOR ADDITIONAL INFORMATION CONTACT

C. W. Bill Young/ DoD Marrow Donor Program
@ 1-800-MARROW-3

Visit our web site @ www.dodmarrow.com

ALL ACTIVE DUTY MILITARY, ACTIVE DUTY DEPENDENTS, DEPARTMENT OF DEFENSE CIVIL SERVICE EMPLOYEES, COAST GUARD, NATIONAL GUARD & DRILLING RESERVE PERSONNEL AGES 18 TO 60 AND IN GOOD HEALTH ARE ELIGIBLE AT NO COST

August of 2002 was a bizarre time for me and it seemed as though chaos and ignorance reigned. A series of incidents left me feeling uncentered, but I soon found my balance again by focusing on the positive and taking action where I could.

August 9, 2002

My good friend and fellow Board member Grace Strong died of lung cancer on August 7th. I was honored to give her eulogy. She was my friend and it was cancer that brought us together. I'll miss our talks about God, family, life, and cancer. Grace gave me the courage to continue with the monument when I wasn't sure if I could take it on and deal with my illness. She said that God was with us and would guide us through.

***

The Allen Cancer Support Group had its own memorial service for Grace. We remembered the time when the group helped her through the tough time of hair loss. We'd all been through it. Hair loss was particularly hard for Grace because she was a lady who went to the beauty salon on a regular basis; her social group existed there. With no hair, Grace felt that she couldn't go to the salon anymore. She missed her friends. She was sad and frustrated that evening and felt like she had no control over her life because of cancer. The support group talked her through it. We brainstormed solutions and finally, we agreed that she didn't have to give up her routine. She could still go to the beauty salon to see her friends, except that she'd wear her wig. It was a simple solution to a big problem, and I'll never forget the brilliance in Grace's face when she realized that she had control back in her life. Grace also went to City Hall with me for one of the first big Foundation presentations made to the City of Allen. For months, our fledging grass-roots committee planned its presentation. Finally the day arrived, and in a crowded room, Grace stood before the Park Board and told them why the monument was important to her. She wanted her great-great grandchildren to know that she was a hero in the War on Cancer. She wanted to give back to the cause so that others might find courage, comfort, enlightenment, and the promise of a cure. Through the legacy of The Cancer Monument, she'd live forever to inspire others.

Grace was weak from chemo that day and she could hardly stand up. Her voice broke from emotion and tears were on many faces. "We need this monument," said Grace. "Help us make it possible for future generations."

As my search for a bone marrow donor went on, near misses and bad news became the norm. From Dallas, the National Marrow Donor Program (NMDP) conducted the international search. We took responsibility too and arranged bone marrow drives through companies and churches in Texas. Stationed in Rhode Island, my brother Ben got the U.S. Navy involved. And since nearly all of my relatives are from the New York area, my family decided to have a huge bone marrow drive on my behalf.

The NMDP didn't operate in New York, another agency did. This particular agency in New York City was the only means by which families in the Hudson Valley, in search of a life-saving donor for a loved one could orchestrate a bone marrow drive.

Back and forth for days, my sister-in-law called to tell me the information that she and my mother received from the Agency Director in Manhattan. I fumed as I listened to the circle of misinformation, outright lies, and double talk they received. I shared the information with my contacts at NMDP in Dallas and there was no other choice but to conclude the unfathomable - the Director of this New York agency was lying to my family, though why, I wasn't sure. As a result, the bone marrow drive in the Newburgh area was prevented. I couldn't imagine why someone would intentionally withhold life-saving information from another in need.

On a mission to fact find, I called the director myself to sort it all out and with one goal in mind; set a date for a bone marrow drive in New York. She proceeded to lie to me too but I was armed with information and knew better. The fact that I was the patient in need of a bone marrow donor made no difference to her. As she continued to throw roadblocks in front of me, her cold tone conveyed the following sentiments: She didn't care. She didn't have cancer. It wasn't her problem. With that, I went full throttle. I no longer felt the need to be business like or civil with a ruthless tyrant and attempted to save my own life over the telephone line.

The angrier I got, the more in charge I became. Low voice. Paced. Authoritative words. I remember only parts of what I said to her. I remember that I told her she was very lucky that I was in Texas and she, in New York; I gave my reasons why and they weren't pretty. I told her that she was an immoral liar and that a cancer diagnosis didn't exclude me the right to have accurate information, respect, or dignity. I said that her efforts to undermine me, and my family, were like a loaded gun to my head and that I didn't take kindly to her death threats.

I asked her to recite her mission statement to me. She stammered. I told her that her personal agenda was unethical and in conflict with her job. I asked for the name and number of her boss. She gave it to me and her tone became friendlier. It was too late. I told her that not only was I going to report her as soon as I hung up the phone, but that her only job that day was to coordinate a bone marrow drive for me by 3:00 p.m.

By the end of day, it was all arranged, I was completely exhausted and a little sad, too. Why did everything have to be so difficult? Joey came home that evening with a bouquet of sunflowers and a grand smile that lifted my spirits. A month later, five hundred people, the Army National Guard and the press attended the bone marrow drive in New York. A community came together for a cause and although no donor matches were found for me, I can't help but believe that as a result of those marrow drives, many lives throughout the world would be saved.

The crisis of cancer brings out the best and the worst in people. I saw this from the beginning of the journey and almost three years later it was no different. One day while I sat in the hospital waiting room, I learned the story of a woman whose abusive husband became even more abusive to her because she needed a bone marrow transplant. After years of isolation within such a marriage, the woman, in her early fifties, no longer felt that she had anyone to help her.

A few years before her leukemia diagnosis, her husband had suffered a stroke and though he'd made a full recovery, he became accustomed to unemployment, and to being waited on hand and foot by his wife. This woman was also one of the millions of people who are self-employed and without health insurance because they can't afford it. Propelled by fear, she somehow managed to still work full time and tend to the every need of her husband, who from his living room recliner, rattled the remaining ice cubes in his glass to signal for a refill.

Once she was on chemo, his brutishness became worse, she told me. He badgered, cursed, name-called, accused her of faking her illness, and told her that her chemo symptoms were "all in her head." I was beyond shock at her story. She was only weeks from receiving a bone marrow transplant, and now actually considered not having the procedure at all. She looked like a shell of a woman imprisoned in a cycle of abuse, but didn't know how to put herself first, even to save her own life.

"Should I have the bone marrow transplant?" she asked me.

I told her how lucky she was to have a donor. She was under the impression that she'd be back at work in a week or two after the transplant until I shared details of my bone marrow experience with her.

"But, I can't be out of work for months. I have to work," she said, "I'm the only household earner." Pale, physically and emotionally drained, her blue eyes looked at me in desperation. "What am I going to do?"

"First, you're going to do whatever it takes to get healthy again," I told her.

"What should I do about my husband?" she asked me.

"Do you really want me to tell you?" I asked.

"Yes," she said with incredible innocence.

I think she was a little shocked at the bluntness of my reply, but by that time, I'd heard enough of outlandish, abusive behavior. I wasn't trying to be nice, I was trying to save her life with a cold splash of reality. Later, it occurred to me that a lot of people probably said the same thing to her at some point and eventually gave up on her. Now, in a life and death crisis, she still couldn't help herself and it pained me to watch a human being spiral downward. Finally, I heard my name called for lab work. I'd been waiting for over ninety minutes and was now one step closer in the process to see my doctor. Before I left this woman, I wrote a series of contacts for her, including the names of social workers, support groups, and how to get on social security.

"Who is your doctor?" I asked her. She told me. "Does he know what you told me here today?" I asked. She hadn't told anyone except me…the stranger in the waiting room. "You should tell a medical person what you told me," I said. "There are social workers, therapists, and resources to help you right here in this hospital. It doesn't have to be this way and it shouldn't be this way at all." She knew it, too. We said our goodbyes and wished each other good luck. Her mouth smiled, but her eyes reflected a lifetime of stress. I never learned her name, or the outcome of her story.

There was the story of two brothers; one in need of a bone marrow donor and the other was his perfect donor match. Within their genes, the family had been given a miracle that most never get and a cure from cancer would seem the likely end to this story. However, these two brothers, for whatever reason, had "bad blood" between them. The great slight was apparently so unforgivable that even the threat of death couldn't create forgiveness and redemption. So, the donor refused to donate marrow to his brother. The act of marrow donation would have required little and would've brought as much pain as a fall on skates. The donor's body would not have been compromised, or at risk in any life threatening way from the small amount of harvested marrow. In fact, new marrow would be made in a day or two. Yet, knowing that his brother had no other options in order to save him from cancer, the man refused to be a marrow donor and his brother died.

Especially for those who've lost loved ones to cancer, coping with the aftermath of death is difficult and unpredictable. This was true for two mothers who became good friends while their children battled leukemia. For a year the families were united in crisis. They prayed together, ate, laughed, and played together at the cancer center. But, when one boy died and the other received a life-saving marrow transplant, the relationship between the mothers became strained with unbearable grief from one, and survivor's guilt from the other to the point that their friendship was no more.

In yet another family story, the crisis of four generations came to a boil when a relative needed a bone marrow transplant. As a result, the skeletons in the family's closet didn't just rattle, they fell out in a big heap of issues that included incest, murder-suicide, child abuse, alcoholism, drug abuse, prison, infidelity, divorce, and more. Decades of violence and tragedy were stuffed in a closet and never healed, or resolved. When the need to find a bone marrow donor arose, already incendiary family bonds exploded. In the process of everyone addressing their own personal crisis and past hurts, the life threatening needs of the person with cancer was compromised to a terrible degree. I never learned the end of that story, but I'd heard enough.

In contrast to these sad stories, there were great and wondrous stories of incredible courage and in one, an entire community came together to raise money and donate their frequent flyer miles so that a family from Africa could travel to America to be tested as a marrow donor for a loved one in need. These stories about successful donor matches filled me with hope that I might find a donor too, and other stories of donor/recipient unions were even more hopeful.

From an expansive genetic pool of millions, a bone marrow match is rare. In a donor search, time is of the essence when cancer cells multiply regularly and the ability of chemo to destroy cancer is not guaranteed. Even if a marrow match is found, there are no guarantees of success. The recipient must be strong enough to endure a transplant. The marrow match must agree to be a donor, be in good health, not pregnant, and with luck, at their last known address in order to be contacted. Beyond gender, age, and cancer type the donor and recipient know nothing about each other.

After a successful transplant, some donors and recipients decide to meet and a few travel across oceans to do so: Three little children hold out a bouquet of flowers and with an unforgettable expression, look into the eyes of the donor from Australia. "Thank you for my mommy," says the oldest child with a soft voice. He doesn't know his alphabet yet, but knows that his parents are happy again and he likes the smell his mother's new hair when he whispers, "I love you" in her ear. Long ago, the donor was unaware that being on the bone marrow registry would make a difference to anyone. He knows differently now. The donor and recipient have waited for this day for over a year and now only tears of gratitude flow as they embrace. The recipient's husband chokes with emotion. He believes in miracles again and shakes the hand of the man he calls "a sweet angel of mercy." With a simple donation of marrow, the donor has restored a family and he thinks to himself; I'd have done more for her if she needed more. He is humbled. He is changed. He will tell this story many times over. For the next fifty years and even to his great grandchildren, he will teach the timeless lesson that one life has the power to change many.

As I prayed that I might receive a marrow donor, I also knew that many people bravely battled cancer and would never receive one. You see, by this time I'd heard many stories about cancer and along the way, came to know a man named Jerry from Michigan. Stephanie courageously battled cancer, and as she waited for a marrow donor that would never come, she held onto hope, her faith, and continued to love everyone around her. I never met Stephanie, but in so many ways her memory inspires me.

Stephanie was the perfect name for an angel so that's what Jerry and Susan named their blonde, blue-eyed daughter who was daddy's little girl from the minute she came into the world. She grew into a beautiful woman who loved to dance so much that her friends nicknamed her "Broadway." After college, she married the man of her dreams, Adam, and became an elementary school teacher. But, one September day everything changed. Stephanie was very sick and two doctor visits resulted in two different diagnoses. The first diagnosis was an ear infection and the other, mononucleosis. She had terrible back pain and was unable to get out of bed. That September also brought the 9-11 tragedy, and while home sick from work that day, Stephanie called her mother to say that she was too weak to even get out of bed to make coffee that morning. Pain and fatigue continued throughout the month until finally, another doctor's opinion was obtained and blood tests were taken.

On October 5th, the ticking clock of a family nightmare began to count down the end of Stephanie's young life. Stephanie had Acute Myelogenous Leukemia (AML). Jerry describes the impact of that news on the family as, "a glass shattering halt." A cancer diagnosis seemed utterly impossible and like many people, Jerry figured that there must have been a mistake at the lab. Cancer happens to other people, he thought, not to us, and certainly not to my beautiful Stephanie. Over the phone, through tears, prayers and careful planning, they vowed to fight together and win the war.

Jerry and Susan lived in Michigan and with the news of Stephanie's cancer they were quickly on a plane to Dallas. Susan gave up her career to become a full-time caregiver for Stephanie. The decision required no deliberation for the sake of their daughter's life, though they didn't realize just how emotionally demanding this role would be.

Jerry said, "Susan witnessed Stephanie's daily battle filled with hopes for the future, courageously fighting to live, and yet, slowly dying every day. To this day, I thank God for Susan, and her unwavering devotion to Stephanie during her illness." Cancer treatments began immediately and Stephanie began her journey into a battle that would forever change her life and the lives of those who so deeply loved her.

Jerry can never forgot the words of his daughter's crying question during the first week of hospitalization. "Dad, why is this happening to me?" she asked. Jerry had no answers and felt helpless. When Stephanie was a little girl, the answers to her questions came so easily and now Jerry couldn't protect her from harm. "I had no answer for why cancer happened to her or anyone else. No one did. The answers would have to come from a higher power, but would we ever truly know why? The only thing I could do was to tell Stephanie how much I loved her and that we'd win the war together. She was a real soldier."

Because Stephanie had AML, she couldn't use her own stem cells for a bone marrow transplant; however, stem cells from a donor's bone marrow could be used instead, and in the majority of cases, offered the chance of success. There were risks too, and one of them was death from organ rejection, known as Graft Versus Host disease. No one in the family was a bone marrow match for Stephanie. The next step in the quest to find an unrelated bone marrow donor involved the search process, but efforts were slowed due to a rare condition that Stephanie had, called Trisomy 8. As the search for a donor continued, Stephanie endured many types of chemo and other drugs to slow down the cancer growth. Just when it looked like she was making progress, the cancer would come back with even more intensity.

The doctors told them about a new drug that filled them with hope. With new marching orders, they prepared for more battle. They were soon in the depths of despair again when it was learned that the procedure couldn't take place; pharmaceutical company restrictions permitted only three patients to receive the drug at a time and the third person had already been chosen. The family was told that they'd "have to wait."

How could they wait? Stephanie was dying and they were running out of options to save her. A few weeks went by, and Stephanie seemed to get better. Jerry flew to Dallas to be with his daughter, wife and son-in law, Adam. He was surprised to see how wonderful Stephanie looked after what she had gone through in the past month.

He reported, 'She seemed so full of strength and spirit and didn't even look sick. We enjoyed the day together and went shopping for a small table for her guest bedroom. Leaving her became increasingly difficult now. I wanted so much to stay with her every day and be a part of her recovery process, but though I couldn't; it was a relief to know that Adam and Susan were with her.'

March turned into April and everything looked positive for Stephanie. No longer required to stay at home due to infection risks, Stephanie was now able to attend church for the first time in many months and reconnected with her friends. The freedom was rewarding for her and Jerry thought that the worst was over. He wondered if God had sent them the miracle that they'd prayed for. Their joy was short-lived and by June, the test results indicated that the Leukemic blasts were at 50%. This time Ara C, Idaurubicin, and Mylotarg were the protocol and the doctors told them that many patients had gone into remission, so they prayed some more. The hard months of battle made Stephanie's body so weak that she could no longer endure any more treatments, though she wanted to still keep up the fight. Without medicine, she couldn't win against cancer. Jerry and Susan prayed that somehow Stephanie's strong personality would override the cancer growth. Of all the times to fly back to Michigan, this was the most difficult for Jerry.

"When will you be back to see me?" Stephanie asked her father.

"How about November? We'll celebrate our birthdays together," he smiled. Jerry knew that Stephanie's time was short, but a part of him refused to acknowledge the worst, for fear that it would become a reality.

"I love you, Sweetheart," he said.

"I love you too, Dad," said Stephanie. They hugged for the last time.

In his story to me titled, "Confessions of a Grieving Father," Jerry writes: "My return home to Grand Rapids was filled with a great deal of crying, screams of anger, and an emotional drain that I had never experienced before in my life. Nothing had any meaning or sense of purpose anymore. During Stephanie's illness, we never spoke of death, only of life and the future. Though I appeared strong on the outside, my heart broke daily with a relentless crushing force and my mind could focus on little else but Stephanie."

A year had passed since Stephanie's diagnosis. One evening, Jerry received word that Stephanie was not responding to respiratory treatments and that she had taken a turn for the worst. He couldn't get a flight to Houston that day, but managed to get one for the next morning. Around 1:30 a.m., the morning of September $4^{th,}$ Jerry awoke to what seemed to be a voice that said, "good-bye." At that moment he knew that his beautiful angel, Stephanie, had passed away and that God was giving him a last moment to say goodbye. Alone in the dark, he imagined Stephanie's beautiful blue eyes and blonde hair as he prayed and said good-bye. Jerry's fears were confirmed when he learned that Stephanie had passed away that morning at 1:30 a.m.

"I cannot explain the amount of grief, pain, and anger I feel today without Stephanie. In time, I know that the grief will subside, but coping through it all is slow and I can't imagine my pain and anger ever going away. I have lost my precious angel, my little girl, and that reality is so completely debilitating that I no longer have the passion for life that I once had. I find myself simply 'going through the motions' on so many days and I am consumed with thoughts of Stephanie. I try to dwell on all the good times we had together, but I am also haunted by memories of the struggles she endured in the last year of her life, and how I as her father was unable to help her."

Throughout her entire battle, Stephanie maintained a high spirit for life and was unwavering in her faith. She wanted to experience motherhood. She wanted to dance and be a teacher again. More than anything she wanted to live. The process of grief is difficult and slow. "My anger is not directed toward God or toward any one individual. I am angry for the loss of Stephanie and for the cancer battle that she so bravely fought, but lost. I am sad that I will never get to hold and kiss her again. I am angry that she never experienced motherhood, the one thing she wanted more than life itself. I will never have a 'Dad's to-do list' from Stephanie again, or feel that great feeling when we'd simply sit and hold hands, or wrap arms, and no words had to be spoken between us. These memories, and a million more, both comfort and sadden me for what I can never have again because of cancer."

"I have been fortunate in my lifetime," Stephanie said to her father one day during his last visit with her.

"Sweetheart, the fortunate ones are those who have been touched by you," he said. Stephanie was loved by so many, and impacted so many lives in her brief thirty-four years.

Jerry writes: "I will never know the Lord's reason for taking her home so soon and can't fathom at this point what that lesson, if any at all, can be. What heavenly significance can there be for us to not to have Stephanie in the world anymore? I've been told by others that, 'some day I will see the beauty of her passing.' Perhaps that is true, but today, I am only at the beginning stages in my journey of grief and coping without my Stephanie. Pain is all that I see, however I do know, and trust, that God will give us direction and guidance through this adversity. My only real comfort and source of coping is the knowledge that Stephanie is now an angel of God. She is whole again and does not suffer any longer. Our family will always honor and celebrate Stephanie's life, and will try to model our lives around the things that were important to her."

***

Cancer forces the range of human emotions whether good or bad, and in a place where I least expected it, more ignorance waited. Another Graduate school semester began and I registered for classes. I still struggled with fatigue issues, so badly that on some days the effort of a phone conversation was just too much. On those days, I'd do nothing at all but rest. Oddly enough, to the general public, although I appeared tired in the months after my failed transplant, I looked healthy. Then, as now, the only way you'd know that I was a cancer survivor was if I told you.

As I sat in the first day of class, the professor read off the rules from the syllabus.

IF YOU MISS A CLASS YOU CAN EXPECT TO FAIL THE COURSE, it said in big black letters. In all my years of academics, I'd never come across such a policy and figured that it was just a scare tactic to weed out the slackers and reduce the large class size. During the fifteen-minute class break, I asked the professor if I could speak to him in private about the policy. For a person with a history of cancer the notion of whether to tell or not is often a vague one. I hadn't been in the habit of announcing my illness to complete strangers but figured that in light of my current health situation a missed class for medical reasons might occur within the next twelve weeks. For the sake of my grade, I wanted to be as up front as possible.

As we stood on the veranda, I informed the professor of my cancer diagnosis. With a long drag of his cigarette, he exhaled his reply. "You have been ill advised to take my class, Ms. Miller. It's unlikely that you can keep pace with the rest of the students. You should go home and take care of yourself." The fact that I'd attended Graduate school for two years with excellent grades while I battled cancer meant nothing to him. "Are you familiar with the term – discrimination?" I asked.

He shuffled his feet, looked across the campus, and was unable to find a way out of the verbal trap he'd fallen into. I dropped his course, found another, and documented the incident in a letter to the Dean as soon as I got home. The next day, I met with the Dean and further reminded him that discrimination lawsuits could bring bad press to a university's reputation. He understood my message. Life went on.

By this time, I had stopped calling the NMDP to find out the latest on donor matches. To this date, no bone marrow donor has ever been found for me. As it neared the end of 2002, I vowed to restore balance to my life in the New Year, regardless of the fact that I still had cancer.

Having cancer was problematic in many ways. At times the unfairness of it all made me a little sad if I thought about it for too long. On such occasions, I'd weigh the facts and reasoned that everyone's life can change in a second because of numerous variables not within our control. I didn't take this cancer journey alone, I told myself, and no one was excluded from the rank and file. Since my diagnosis in March 2000, millions of Americans had been newly diagnosed with cancer and if you weren't one of the diagnosed, chances were that you knew someone who was. In either case, a nation was affected. I considered the fact that millions of undiagnosed people walk around with cancer. Still too small to be detected, cancer waits to strike them while they live under the assumption of good health. In a few more years, their lives and the lives of their loved ones will change forever because of cancer.

That had been my reality. Life with cancer wasn't preferable, but it could be much worse, I thought. At least I have the benefit of knowledge, I'd think. Okay, I'd reason, science can't cure me at the moment, but there's an answer out there with my name all over it. I'll focus on living and prepare for the cancer battle ahead. On these occasions when I'd balance the facts against philosophy and emotion, I'd remember the woman on the Greek island that I met a decade earlier and was thankful to now stand naked and bruised in the truth instead of cloaked in ignorance. Ignorance is never bliss I'd think it's just downright stupid.

Eight months after my bone marrow transplant, chemo-related fatigue still ruled my every waking moment and all energy spurts were used up as quickly as they came. Days on the couch with a remote control were preferable, but the monument was full speed ahead. Public appearances in triple-digit temperatures, constant planning, endless writing, talking, and meetings on its behalf had become a full-time endeavor.

Gosh, I'd think, I'm not running for Congress, I'm just trying to build a monument! Public opinion for the monument inspired me onward and no matter what group I spoke to: a city council, a church, a cancer support group, or a community group, the consensus was the same – The Cancer Monument was wanted and needed. I learned the stories of those who needed the monument most: children like Kaitlyn, Olivia, and Hannah who are too young yet to know about cancer, but who will one day learn of the heroism of a grandparent, or great-grandparent that battled in the War on Cancer. There were people like Audrey, an oncology nurse whose father died of cancer years earlier when she was in high school. Audrey's dad once built a magnificent fireplace in the family's home. Brick by brick, Audrey watched her father build the fireplace, which became a happy focal point for everyone. Many photos were taken in front of that fireplace, many stories told, many plans made, and holidays celebrated. When Audrey's father died, the fireplace became a symbolic place to remember him and on days when she wasn't able to visit his grave, she'd sit on the red brick hearth and talk to him. Sometimes, she'd hold her body against the bricks and spread her arms across the length of it as if to embrace her father once again. He'd once been there to breathe the air in that room. He had loved them all. He had touched every single brick.

The year that her dad died, Audrey went away to college, and that Christmas, the weather was too snowy to travel home. Alone in a cemetery on Christmas, Audrey sat at the grave of a stranger, touched the headstone, and talked out loud to her father as though she were seated beside the living room fireplace he'd built. When Audrey told me her story I was speechless. We'd been discussing what The Cancer Monument would mean to her.

"For me, the monument is like that fireplace, a way of being close to my father, and a way to keep his memory alive. To know that there are other people at the monument to cope, grieve, and celebrate their loved ones will bond us; it'll be like a ready made support group to share our stories."

***

One day in the frozen food aisle of my local supermarket, I was reminded again about the need for continuous support when I bumped into Donna and her children. I hadn't seen her since before my transplant and when she asked me how I was, I let her know that my cancer was back. She was a breast cancer survivor and two years in remission. With my news of re-occurrence, her fears rippled into a wave of terror. Her tears flowed with the memories of surgery, chemo, and the entire episode flashed before her as though it were happening all over again. She smelled the alcohol pads and envisioned her doctor's office as she stood next to the frozen pizza at the grocery store. Her teenaged daughter assured her that she'd be okay as her two younger children occupied themselves with some made-up game further down the aisle.

"I don't know what I'll do if it comes back again," she said.

"You'll put one foot in front of the other and fight," I said.

"How can you be so positive when you still have cancer?" she asked me.

"Today I'm positive, tomorrow I might not be," I laughed. "It's a process. Besides, you have the best motivation of all," I said, and pointed to her children.

***

Our constituency had measurably grown by the end of 2002 and The Cancer Monument positioned for large-scale efforts to gather the 60,000 Honoree names that would be inscribed to fund its construction. At the same time, negotiations were underway with the City of Allen, which would define the legal process and designate a piece of parkland to become the monument's home. The process of politics and bureaucracy was too slow for my liking, but in the City of Allen's fifty years, no charitable organization had ever wanted to build and donate such a public monument. No matter the pace, a system of checks and balances was required and only a job well done would matter in the end.

For all of my impatience, everything was coming together and a burgeoning national public sentiment revealed the following about our Honored Heroes:

"My children were just babies when I battled cancer; they don't remember that scary time when our family was turned upside down. The Cancer Monument will make it easier to tell them the story and teach them about cancer, too. I can't wait to take my entire family to The Cancer Monument." David – Michigan

***

"Justin was only 7 years old when he battled cancer, but his bravery inspired us all." Ginger – Texas

***

"Our family is spread across the country and has been hit by cancer many times over. The Cancer Monument gives us a place to remember and honor them all." The Dean Family – Ohio

***

The people had spoken. They understood the monument's concepts and it was a part of their hearts and minds. Though we hadn't officially kicked off our "Who's Your Hero" name-gathering campaign yet, the message of the monument's arrival spread by word of mouth and generated Honoree names. I was thrilled to see every Honoree inscription form. They came from Alaska, Oklahoma, Florida, Michigan, New York, Connecticut, California and many other states. But, there was still a lot more work to do before 60,000 names would be obtained.

On the eve of 2003, I vowed to be in pursuit of two things for the New Year: Exercise and Fun! I threw out the shower bench even though I still needed it and bought a treadmill instead. I was terribly out of shape and couldn't get through a four-minute walk on snail speed. So, I hired a personal trainer who'd help motivate me. My old trainer was now in another profession, but my friend Rebecca had raved about her personal trainer, Shawn Osmond. After several months of muscle rebuilding and cardiovascular work with Shawn, I was able to do a light jog on an incline.

By the end of the summer it felt like the old days back at the gym. Three times a week I ran, curled biceps, crunched abs and deep knee squatted with an exercise ball for one-hour sessions with Shawn. We'd laugh, talk, and exercise at the same time. I'd drip with sweat and felt as though my cells screamed out victory for themselves, "Yahooo!" There were definitely times when I did too.

"I'm back, I'm back!" I'd exclaim to Shawn as I ran on the treadmill.

"Yes, you are!" she'd say.

"You can't keep me down cancer...there...take that..." I'd say and burst into a full speed run as though I could mow cancer down.

As the months went by with no cancer treatments, physically I became stronger. At times, I had to remind myself that I still had cancer. For my sanity, I completely stopped my inquiries about a bone marrow donor though the search for one still continued. I figured if there were any worthwhile news, I'd hear about it. The fact that I continued to have cancer with no cure in sight was a reality difficult enough, but to make myself wear the heavy burden of it around my neck like a noose every second of every day would have prevented quality living.

I reminded myself that it was my duty and obligation to focus on making a life with the possibility of no cure. Hope. Faith. Though these words were at times a little battered, there was a core strength in them that couldn't be ignored. I planted flowers that year and took walks in the park with Joey and Buddy. I met Mike and Gloria in Vegas and with the wind in my hair and rock music blaring in my ears I sped down Las Vegas Boulevard in a red Mustang convertible. I flew over the Grand Canyon in a helicopter and though it was a magnificent sight, it was scary as hell and vowed that I'd never do it again.

I took a trip to Manhattan that summer and was joined by Mike, Ben, Gloria, and my little nephew. I had missed walking in a crowded, noisy street. I missed the people, the slang and the thick New York accent, which was comfortably my own. Though I lived in Texas for five years, a word or two still gave away the fact that I was from somewhere north. I missed the entire vibe of the city. It was a part of me, every bit of it: Rockefeller Center, St. Patrick's Cathedral, Greenwich Village, the glorious storefront windows, the pretzel vendors, sidewalk artists, traffic, summer heat, and even the puffs of white steam that rose from the sewers.

We hardly slept that trip and mostly ate our way through New York: Gelato and Clams Casino in Little Italy, six inches of Lox and Bagels at the Carnegie Deli, sushi somewhere uptown, a bowl of cherries at the Plaza Hotel, room service at the Waldorf, and the impeccable experience of an 1863 Madeira wine at a 5th Avenue French restaurant. All of which made me forget for a while that I had no cancer treatment options available to me. My nephew's excitement over all the toys at FAO Schwartz, and the playful seals at the Central Park Zoo made me feel like a kid again. We took a horse drawn carriage ride through Central Park just like I imagined during the long days of my transplant more than a year earlier. We walked beside the flowered pond to see the ducks and sat on a bench under the cool shade to watch a juggler. We decided not to go to the site where the Twin Towers once stood; we wanted to remember it as we'd experienced it. Magnificent. Proud.

Another set of P.E.T. scans revealed an oddity that summer. My cancer cells had shrunk.

"Whatever you're doing, keep doing it!" said Dr. Agura. He paused and with curiosity he asked me, "What are you doing?"

"I'm happy," I said.

***

That summer meeting with Dr. Agura brought new information and hope to Joey and me about the next step in my cancer treatment plan. We learned about an immunotherapy drug called Rituxan. It had made its way to FDA approval and in clinical trials had shown remarkable results in sustained remissions for Non-Hodgkin's Lymphoma cases. The years of clinical trials and subsequent patient progress reports told one successful cancer story after another because of Rituxan. New information suggested that the drug could be successfully used for Hodgkin's Lymphoma case like my own.

Unlike chemotherapy, Rituxan has no side effects except for maybe some flu-like symptoms Dr. Agura described. Compared to chemo, the flu sounded like a fun time. With Rituxan there'd be no down time or a long recovery period afterward. This type of cancer treatment sounded like rainbows, lollipops, and the stuff of science fiction. No suffering? Could it be true? The technology of Rituxan was designed to target and destroy existing cancer cells within the body. Dr. Agura was full of smiles when he talked about even more immunotherapy drugs that were soon to become available because of research. Immunotherapy drugs promised cures and a whole new way of cancer treatment that would restore hope, and a quality of life back to patient and family.

There was one problem however, Rituxan was very expensive and my health insurance provider wouldn't pay for the treatments. I felt dejected. In a split second I was ready to give up, tired of fighting to stay alive. My hope to be cured of cancer fell through my fingers like sand.

"We'll fight the insurance company," Dr. Agura said. "I have enough information to make your case. They'll have to say yes. It may take a while but we have to try." At the doctor's confident words my fire was re-ignited and I resigned to tear the enemy apart on a new battlefield.

Then, a week later I learned about a lecture on clinical trials being given by Dr. Wendy Harpham. Dr. Harpham, a medical doctor and mother of three children, is also a cancer survivor who battled Non-Hodgkin's Lymphoma for eight years before she found a treatment that gave her a lasting remission. The details of that journey I didn't know until the evening of her lecture. I'd already read Dr. Harpham's book, After Cancer. A friend gave me an autographed copy a year earlier when my cancer returned. On the day of Dr. Harpham's lecture I struggled with fatigue and low spirits. Though Dr. Agura's determination to persist with my insurance company invigorated me to stay in the fight, I sometimes felt trapped by my illness. My mind was free, my body was sick, and I lived in a world that abided by a bureaucratic process.

I wondered if cancer would kill me before I'd ever be approved for Rituxan. Maybe like my stem cell transplant, it wouldn't even work. Aside from that, who was I to the insurance company anyway? At times, I imagined some emperor-like decision-making process: Thumbs up, she lives. Thumbs down, she dies. The way I saw it, to the insurance company I was just some costly nobody with cancer and one of hundreds of faceless files that cluttered someone's office cubicle. My life was in the hands of a stranger at an insurance office, and I didn't like it one bit. If there was hope to be found in my situation I couldn't find it that afternoon.

Just when I'd resigned myself to laying on the couch with a remote control, the telephone rang.

"Hi, I'm just calling to remind you about Dr. Harpham's lecture this evening."

"I have the book," I said with an abrupt tone.

"No, no, the voice on the phone said, you have to come." " Promise me."

"Okay," I said with a softer voice. "I'll be there." There was something about the caller's determined tone that pulled me out of my emotional funk, and suddenly I was getting ready to attend a lecture instead of watching re-runs of Seinfeld.

Dr. Harpham's cancer battle began in 1990. After several cancer therapies like chemo, radiation, and Interferon that gave her short remissions, the opportunity to participate in a clinical trial for a new immunotherapy drug was an option that she chose. It was Rituxan! I couldn't believe my ears as I watched the healthy, vital-appearing woman behind the microphone.

Dr. Harpham explained that in 1993 she was one of fifteen pioneering patients in the Phase I trial of Rituxan, then called IDEC-

C2B8. By 1998 she'd receive a total of four rounds. More than a decade had passed since her first diagnosis. The expression of that time was perfectly captured in the slide presentation, which included family photos of her children who, only babies when when she was diagnosed, were now all teenagers. Because of Rituxan, Dr. Harpham has been cancer-free and writing more books ever since. Inspired by Dr. Harpham's determination, I wanted my dose of Rituxan too. I wanted to achieve so many things including motherhood, but unless I was cancer-free that wouldn't be possible. Because of my insurance company, my chance for a cancer-free life was on hold.

In the meantime, work in the community for The Cancer Monument continued and I felt fulfilled every time I saw the look of wonder on the face of someone who couldn't believe that such a structure was intended to celebrate their heroism. The Heroes came in all varieties: a fourteen-year-old boy with leukemia, a seven-year lung cancer survivor, a brain cancer survivor who held his newborn daughter, people with stomach cancer, pancreatic, breast cancer, children, grandparents, everyone had cancer. Some had lost their battles, some still battled, and others had won. As we campaigned for the Honoree names that would build the monument, we educated the public on a variety of topics along the way including: anti-tobacco, skin cancer awareness, colon cancer awareness, and the bone marrow donor registry. The Cancer Monument provided an open forum to discuss all cancer types and though the monument wasn't built yet, it was already doing the job that was intended.

Soon we had public support in 20 states and testimonials like these say it all:

"My mom died of cancer when I was 5 years old...I was one of the very few children that didn't have a mom and there was certainly no mom to wish a happy Mother's Day...The Cancer Monument will be a tangible way for me to honor my mother and it will be a comfort to know that others will have an opportunity to honor their loved ones also." — Debe in Texas

***

"This monument gives my family and I the opportunity to remember my grandmother in a way that will last a lifetime. Her name along with countless others will be etched in stone. My children's children will have the opportunity to visit a serene site where they can see the impact of this place and the countless lives touched. You are putting a name on the infinite that pass unnoticed and giving a voice for those losing, winning, and struggling with this battle. God Bless!" —Heather

***

"Being a two-time cancer survivor, I have met many people whose lives have been affected by cancer. I have met those going through their battle and I have met those that watched a loved one go through the battle. Some were lucky enough to be called 'survivors' such as myself. Others weren't so lucky. They are no longer here to speak to, to hug, or to brighten someone's day, but they will never be forgotten. Thanks to The Cancer Monument they will be honored and remembered. I feel very fortunate to live so close to where the monument is being built. I will be able to reflect upon my surviving sisters and brothers of cancer and have a place to talk to those that lost their battle, as well as a place to stop and reflect about my journey!" — Kathey

***

"This monument is the first of its kind for those touched by cancer. It will create conversations, awareness and education. What a wonderful gift to the community." — The American Cancer Society - Allen Magazine, November 2002

***

"You do not lose your Heroes just because you are no longer able to touch them. They are still with you – giving you strength, courage and advice just as they did every other day of your life. Our Heroes are the two most amazing people we ever knew, our parents, and we can only hope to be as brave and selfless as they were when the demon known as cancer attacked them without notice. The Cancer Monument's fight gives us all the realization that a cure will be found sometime in the future. It is the type of courage and desire that is shown by all of the victims and survivors of cancer – the true Heroes in today's world. These are the thousands of people represented. For without the brave fight demonstrated by our Heroes, there is no victory and this is one challenge that we will overcome." — Lisa

***

"The Cancer Monument will be a physical place where I can not only honor my mother by inscribing her name, but can also reflect on memories of her while surrounded by the beauty of this magnificent monument which is so symbolic of life, past, present, and future. This enormous undertaking has filled me with feelings of pride, wonder, understanding, hope, anticipation, expectation, and so much more. I am inspired to be a better person and to not give up so easily, especially when you know that what you are doing is right and good." — Vickie

***

"Knowing that there is a movement, and a project dedicated to cancer 'heroes' brightens my heart. The journey that these individuals must endure is monumental, and to reward that journey with The Cancer Monument is a great symbol of hope, friendship, and love. For my wife and I, The Cancer Monument will represent one of the many bright 'lights' that will continue to shine for our daughter, Stephanie."
—Jerry in Michigan

***

"The Cancer Monument has been and will always be an inspiration for those of us 'left behind' from the effects of cancer." — Sandy

***

By November, things were in high gear. Even though I still had cancer, Joey and I decided not to prevent our family planning endeavors and took steps to investigate our options. We looked into a variety of choices and for us, foreign adoption provided the best of all possible scenarios and the least amount of legal ambiguity once a child was placed into our custody. For two years, we interviewed adoption agencies, scoured through websites and brochures, attended workshops and met a number of parents and children who'd made successful, happy families with adoptions in China and Russia. The children were adorable, bright, articulate, and no matter their country of birth, they were now American kids through and through.

After leaving an adoption family reunion, hosted by an agency one autumn day, I was undecided about whether to choose a boy, a girl and from which country. As we drove home I asked Joey, "When you imagine our family, what do you see? Do you see a child from China, Russia, or maybe even Haiti or South America? What does our family look like in your mind?" I felt curious anticipation.

"Happy. Our family looks happy," Joey said.

"Let's make a nursery," I said. "If you build it he will come. Right? It'll be our torch of progress because if we can adopt a child, then that means I'm cancer-free." So, we bought a crib and some other baby furniture along with a few outfits and every now and then I'd pretend that a little happy face waited for me inside that room.

***

The details of the contract with the City of Allen were still being ironed out, but a building site for the monument had been selected and that November 2003, we had a dedication ceremony. It was a day that I'll never forget. That morning, cancer survivors, city officials from Allen, members of the clergy, media, and the medical profession joined in music, prayer, and heartfelt speeches. We commemorated the importance of that day and looked forward to the monument that would one day stand there with the force of 60,000 Hero names upon it.

Along with a cancer diagnosis can come shame, fear, despair, and the stigma of victimization. The Cancer Monument is unconventional weaponry. It replaces negativity with hope, education, the promise of a cure, and needed inspiration gained from the more assertive philosophy that we are gallant, soldier-heroes in a War on Cancer. To a cancer patient, this viewpoint of honor and distinction can mean the difference between continuing to cope and fight, or not. These very concepts of the Monument were repeated again that day in front of the community as a confirmation that we were on our way to seeing it built one day soon.

My friend, Mary Ann, also spoke that day; she'd been in the battle against Non-Hodgkins' Lymphoma for several years. Mary Ann had a zany sense of humor and wore crazy hats just to keep the mood light.

"Cancer requires laughter, don't you think?" she asked me one day. But, that day, Mary Ann put jokes aside and spoke on behalf of all who battled cancer and even for those in heaven who could no longer be heard. Her closing words sent a shiver up my spine. Slow and succinct she said, "Do not forget us." Six months later, she was dead.

December brought bittersweet news. My youngest brother, Shaun, was engaged to a young woman named Cari he'd met in the military while stationed in Germany. That was the good part. Cari, a West Point graduate, had recently received orders to be sent to the war in Iraq. In love, my brother requested an Army transfer to go to Iraq also. As the months of beheadings and roadside bombs increased in the Middle East, I felt sure that stress would cause new forms of cancer for me. Shaun's emails to me couldn't reveal much about his location, or duties. As his sister, I didn't care if he wrote the alphabet to me, so long as I heard from him.

In one email he wrote: "All is well here. Getting pretty hot though still in 110 to 120 degree temperatures. Can't take this heat. Heck, I'm from New York where it snows eight months a year. I pray that not only do you win your own battle, but that we do, too, over here and that we are all able to walk away from it and be safe again back home." Love, your brother Shaun

***

Meanwhile, I graduated with a Masters degree in Humanities-Literature with a 3.75 grade point average and was accepted into the Ph.D. program in Public Affairs at The University of Texas at Dallas and also found out that month that my cancer had grown to a size that required me to go back on chemotherapy. I was long past tears over cancer and just trying to get on with life. The good news was that this chemo regimen didn't cause my hair to fall out and was mostly in pill form. But the rest of the chemo biz was the same: low blood counts, dizziness, fatigue, bruising, blood transfusions, shortness of breath, and a long list of other side effects. I was in the trenches again.

My workouts stopped, and for eight more months I couldn't exercise. This time, I refused to buy another shower bench and instead, I sat on Santa's lap that December, and half joked when I told him that my wish was to be cancer-free. His elves couldn't make that holiday dream come true, but Santa did say that he'd send his prayers right up to heaven for me.

By May, I managed to finish my first semester of Ph.D. work with perfect grades, and Dr. Agura's persistence with my insurance company resulted in an approval letter for Rituxan. As I held the approval letter in my hand, a great sense of victory came over me. Maybe I'd beat cancer after all, I thought. As soon as I was in remission, eight treatments of Rituxan would have my name written all over them. My cancer was brought under control, and by late June the P.E.T. scan indicated no cancer. The fact that I was in remission was a thrill, but without the help of advanced cancer therapies like Rituxan, it wasn't likely to last.

***

<u>July 23, 2004</u>

Yesterday was my 38th birthday. I had my first treatment of Rituxan today and will have seven more on a weekly basis. The drug was given through an I.V. drip that lasted several hours. I experienced no side effects. Rituxan is made from mice. I wonder if I'll crave lots of cheese. Ha-Ha!

August 10, 2004

Joey had his braces removed today. His smile brightens my day.

September 10, 2004

Today was my last treatment of Rituxan. I have completed eight doses and will have a P.E.T. scan on the 24th that will tell whether I am still in remission. If so, I'll continue to be monitored as the months and years go by. If cancer returns, we'll find another plan. In either case, I do not fear cancer. I disembowel its power by living fully, in spite of it, and I will always be ready for the fight. I said goodbye to my illness and hello to health. Ironically, 4:00 p.m. was the hour of my birth. Today, it is the hour of my re-birth. Hello world! Hello to goodness, inner peace, and a balanced life. Hello to wisdom, joy, purpose, and truth.

Now, after years of hard work, the elements are in place to build The Cancer Monument and the only thing needed is 60,000 Honoree names. The contract was signed with the City of Allen in July. It allocates two acres of property for the monument and gives us the next five years to obtain our 60,000 names so that we can fund the project and build. At this point, it's up to the public now to support our mission. They must seize the opportunity while it is still available, and submit inscription forms on behalf of their Honored Heroes. In the years ahead, I will lead the Foundation in its mission. This is the last entry of my cancer journal. I have begun a new one – an adoption journal and with it, the inspiration of a book about adoption after cancer. For Joey and me, adoption brings the promise of a new beginning: an orphaned child in a far away land is in need of parents and we are parents, in need of a child. The hand of God will bring us all together one day soon.

***

As 2004 draws to a close, there is much to be thankful for. I am cancer-free. To date, The Cancer Monument has received Hero names from 20 states. We are on our way to achieve our goal of 60,000 names. Once all names are received, we'll begin construction. I'm writing three more books and hosting a new radio program called Monumental People Coping and Living With Cancer. On the personal side, Joey and I will begin the New Year with a renewal of our wedding vows on the island of Jamaica where we were to be married almost five years ago.

My recovery from years of cancer treatments is slow and fatigue is an unpredictable, daily issue. Because of cancer treatments, secondary cancers and organ deterioration are possible whether twenty, or fifty years from now, or maybe never. If necessary, I'll always be ready to war against cancer. I am proud to be a cancer survivor.

I know there are many real challenges ahead. My duty as a survivor is to live a healthy, happy, and purposeful life. I can't predict the future, but Joey and I embrace our lives as fate intends for it to be. I'm still discovering my self-concept, body image, and my feminine worth. I now remind myself that self-acceptance is a process. With that, I feel a little wiser. I'm long past the days of the coordinated purse and shoes requirement. I've let go of a lot of misconceptions like that, thanks to my cancer battle.

Our spare bedroom is now a nursery and with great excitement, Joey and I prepare to be parents. Now that I'm cancer-free, I've begun a newer journey, which includes motherhood and adoption after cancer. The topic of adoption after cancer is one with many issues and obstacles. This new life journey is also the subject of another book that I am writing, which will include excerpts from my private adoption journal that I keep for myself, and for the son that we've already named Nicholas.

Adoption Journal Excerpts: Letters To Nicholas

<u>October 17, 2004</u>
Dear Nicholas,

I am your mother. Though I am not the woman to whom you were born, I am the woman that God intends to love, protect and show you the way to a joyful and purposeful life. I am married to a wonderful man who will be your father. His name is Joey and like me, his eyes fill with tears whenever we talk about you. You are the child of our hearts. It is likely that at the time of this letter you have not yet been born though your presence is already felt here on earth. We chose your name more than a year ago and now there is a nursery that waits for you in our home. I walk inside your room on many days and try to imagine your beautiful face and outstretched arms that will one day embrace me and call me mommy.

The story of how you will come into the world to first become an orphan in Russia is a long one with many details and through the years you will come to know it as we do. Though your life began with adversity, much love and opportunity waits for you with us in America.

You will also know one day about the many people who are right now a part of your life story and are helping in the process to bring you home. Much of the details of your life before you entered the orphanage will not be available because of the closed adoption records and laws in Russia. Chances are, I will not know about your biological family and why they gave you up. I can only imagine that their decision was very difficult and that they loved you enough to do so and will think about you every day with as much passion as we think about you now. I have begun the process of writing this journal for you and for me too so that one day when you are filled with many questions about yourself in this world, it will serve to help you understand, to make you proud, and rejoice in who you are.

***

October 22, 2004

Dear Nicholas,

For many reasons there are people who are unable to have biologic children. Some people cannot have children because they battled a disease called cancer and the medicines that they took to be healthy again made them infertile. I am one of those people. As you will learn through the years, life is a mixture of adversity and victories, but what we can take away from each experience are lessons that make us better people. You will also come to understand that being a parent requires more than biology alone. We are your parents because we are committed to the well-being of your life. We are guided by love in our hearts for you.

Your father and I planned to have children once we were married. We talked about marriage and family on our very first date in January 1997. We wanted a boy and a girl. However, Fate stepped in and two months before our wedding I was diagnosed with cancer. That was in March 2000. I was only 33 years old. Cancer changed our lives in many positive ways and we've been able to help many people throughout the world because of it, however, as a result of medicines that I took to be cured, my ovaries were destroyed and I became unable to have biologic children. Nicholas, as you become a young man you will learn that sometimes God provides the only consolation for us when tragedy strikes. When there are no logical reasons and unfairness seems insurmountable, please always remember that God loves you and even though bad things may happen, He has a plan for you. This is the philosophy that your Daddy and I have accepted as the reason why we can no longer havebiologic children. The course of events that have happened to us is God's will because He had a better plan for us. I am grateful to have survived cancer. If I didn't have cancer, it is unlikely that we would ever be your parents at all. Nicholas, you should never question for one moment how wanted and purposeful you are in this world. Though you may not even be born yet, already, you are a great teacher and have given us the gift of hope.

***

October 29, 2004

Dear Nicholas,

I bought some puzzles and books for you today. The books are from the Winnie the Pooh series and the puzzles will help you learn your numbers, letters and the map of the United States. I can't wait to teach you how to read and write. Maybe you'd like to be a doctor or a scientist when you grow up!

***

November 3, 2004

Dear Nicholas,

Last night your Daddy and I stood inside your nursery and thought about you. The time is fast approaching that we will be together soon. Already we love you, though we have not met you yet. You are our hope and prayer. I feel that the angels are at work to make it all possible. There are challenges ahead, but with cancer behind me now, these are the happy times. In the happy times, no one is in the search for answers. Through the stages of your life, you will ask 'why' about so many things and that is good. Always be on the search for answers. Be honorable and kind. Be a person of action, defend the weak, and do not be persuaded by the unjust.

As your parents, we will guide you and help to build your character so that you may stand firmly in this world, make your own decisions, and carry out your personal mission for being here. Nicholas, when there are no earthly answers for your troubles and burdens, you must take comfort in the protective knowledge that the answers you seek are in the hands of God and will one day be revealed to you in His measure of time.

Prevention
Awareness
Resources

Cancer Prevention and Awareness Information

- According to the National Foundation for Cancer Research, you should consult your doctor for a thorough check-up if you display any of the following symptoms: change in bowel or bladder habits; a sore that does not heal; unusual bleeding or discharge; thickening or lumps in breast or elsewhere; indigestion or difficulty swallowing; obvious change in wart or mole; nagging cough or hoarseness; persistent aching.
- According to both the National Foundation for Cancer Research and the American Institute for Cancer Research, nutrition is your best prevention against cancer. Research shows that as many as one-third of all cancers are the result of a poor diet low in fruits, vegetables and lean proteins.
- Due to cancer prevention efforts and cancer education, tobacco use among high school students dropped almost 22 percent in 2003; according to the Centers for Disease Control and Prevention, this is the lowest level in more than 10 years.
- Breast cancer can be detected early with mammography, clinical breast exams and also breast self-exams. Generally, women aged 40-50 should have a mammogram every year, but those with a family history of breast cancer should consider earlier screenings. Talk to your physician about what is right for you. Symptoms to report to your doctor are: a lump or thickening in the breast or armpit, a change in the color of the breast, discharge, skin texture or other abnormalities. Just because you are not yet 40 doesn't mean that you can't get breast cancer. Women in their 20s get breast cancer, too. Men can also get breast cancer.
- There is a greater risk of cervical cancer among women who had sex at an early age, multiple sexual partners, a history of the human papilloma virus (HPV), or who have had more than five pregnancies. One of the ways to prevent cervical cancer is to practice safe sex, because it reduces your exposure to

sexually transmitted diseases. Using a barrier method of birth control, such as a condom or having sex with only one long-term partner, also can reduce your exposure to these diseases. Regular screening tests, including a pelvic examination and Pap test, can detect changes in cervical cells before they have an opportunity to become cancerous.

- A family history of cancer can increase your risk for developing cancer. A family history contributes a risk factor for some of the common cancers, including: breast, colon, ovarian, and prostate.

- Population studies have found a direct correlation between diet and the development of esophageal cancer. Diets low in beta-carotene, vitamins A, C, B, magnesium, and zinc have been associated with cancer. Also, reduced consumption of fruits, vegetables, fresh meat, fresh fish and dairy products resulted in a 2-fold increased incidence of esophageal carcinoma.

- High-level exposure to asbestos, ionizing radiation, and drinking exceptionally hot beverages like tea has been correlated to esophageal carcinomas.

- Smoking and alcohol drinking are the two major factors of esophageal carcinomas. Second hand smoke increases the risk of cancer for others who do not smoke. Cigars, pipes or chewing tobacco is not safe smoking. No tobacco products are safe.

- Screening for colorectal cancer should be offered to all men and women without risk factors, beginning at age 50. Embarrassment often plays a role in avoiding screening exams for colorectal cancer. The vast majority of colon cancers can occur in people who have no identified risk factors and can occur in people as in their 20s and 30s. The greatest impact made against colon cancer is early detection made with screenings, which detect polyps or to find cancers at a very early stage so that they can be surgically removed before spreading occurs.

- Grilling foods may raise the risk of cancer, but following a few guidelines for safer grilling can reduce that risk. The longer food stays on the grill, the more HAA-carcinogens are formed which may increase cancer risk. By taking a few precautions, you can minimize the cancer risk and still enjoy cookouts: Reduce fat drippings by selecting low-fat cuts of meat; trim away excess fat and remove poultry skin; marinate meat; reduce grilling time by precooking meats; do not char, or eat any portion of the meat that is charred.

- There is no such thing as a "safe" tan. Tanning beds will not prevent cancer. Sun-protective clothes block out harmful ultraviolet sunrays or UV rays. Sun protective clothes are darker, have a tighter weave or knit than traditional fabrics and are labeled with an Ultraviolet Protection Factor (UPF).

- Avoid unnecessary sun exposure, especially between 10:00 a.m. and 4:00 p.m., the peak hours for harmful ultraviolet (UV) radiation. When outdoors, use sunscreens rated SPF 15 or higher. Apply them liberally, and frequently. Cover up when exposed to sunlight; also wear hat and UV-protective sunglasses.

- Teach your children good sun protection habits at an early age: The damage that leads to adult skin cancers starts in childhood. Examine your skin at least once every three months for any strange moles and if found, consult with your doctor.

- Don't forget that the sun's harmful ultraviolet (UV) radiation can also go through automobile and residential windows, which can also contribute to cataracts, macular degeneration, and eyelid cancers. When you're on snow or ice, your face and eyes are at almost twice the risk of UV damage because of reflected glare.

- Cancer is not contagious.

- There is no scientific data to show that stress causes cancer.

- Studies have found that risk factors for pancreatic cancer increase with age, smoking, diabetes, being male, chronic pancreatitis, or a family history of pancreatic cancers.

- According to the National Cancer Institute, the chance of

getting prostate cancer goes up sharply as a man gets older. In the U.S., most men with prostate cancer are older than 65.

- For more information about thyroid cancer or go to www.thyca.org.

- Most brain tumors are detected in people who are 70 years old or older. However, brain tumors are the second most common cancer in children and more common in children younger than 8-years-old.

- If you are a caregiver to someone with cancer, remember to take care of yourself. Caregivers can find support by attending a support group. Ask your doctor, nurse, or local church for the nearest cancer support group.

Additional Resource Information

Cancer Together
http://www.cancertogether.org

Capital of Texas Team Survivor:
P.O. Box 301148
Austin, Texas 78703-0020
http://www.teamsurvivoraustin.org

City of Allen Animal Shelter:
770 S. Allen Heights Drive,
Allen, Texas 75002; 972-727-0230
http://www.perfinder.org

Labrador Retriever Rescue of North Texas:
972-480-LABS (5227)
http://www.labrescuenorthtexas.org

National Marrow Donor Program
http://www.marrow.org

The National Center for Complementary and Alternative Medicine (NCCAM)
http://nccam.nih.gov

The Stephanie Robinson Foundation:
C/O The Dallas Foundation, 900 Jackson St. Suite 150,
Dallas, Texas 75202

Who's Your Hero?

Visit http://www.TheCancerMonument.org to obtain inscription forms.

Honor your Hero in the War on Cancer today and let's build The Cancer Monument!

About The Author

Michelle Miller is a cancer survivor and Founding President of The Cancer Monument Incorporated a non-profit charitable 501c3 organization. As visionary and creator of The Cancer Monument, a nationally awaited monument in the making, Michelle is an advocate for cancer research, prevention and awareness. She is earning a Ph.D. in Public Affairs at The State University of Texas at Dallas. She holds an M.A. in Humanities-Literature, with a B.A. in English Literature from the State University of New York at Stony Brook. She currently authors other books including: Dog Tales-Cancer Stories For Kids, Voices From The War On Cancer, and Journey From Cancer To Adoption, part of the P.A.R.Q. Cancer Education Series. A member of the Society of Children's Book Writers and Illustrators and National Association of Women Writers, Michelle's newspaper column, Surviving Cancer, appeared in Dallas/Fort Worth community papers in 2001. Michelle has been a frequent guest of Texas radio and television as well as a guest speaker and free-lance writer for several cancer organizations. A member of the National Association of Broadcasters, Miller is the producer, writer, and host of Monumental People Coping and Living With Cancer, a public service educational radio forum. A native New Yorker who makes her home in the Dallas area since 1998, Michelle lives with her husband Joey and their Black Labrador Retriever, "Buddy The Wonder Dog." She can be reached through her Foundation website at http://www.thecancermonument.org.

Other Contributors:

Sabra King is a Dallas based free-lance writer and poet. She is the Founder and owner of Paper Canvas, a company that offers creative and technical writing services. She also serves as Vice President of Publishing and Editor-in-Chief of RED Magazine, a Prime Demographics lifestyle publication. Sabra serves on the Board of Directors for The Cancer Monument Incorporated as Director of Fundraising and Events. She can be reached through the Foundation at Sabra.King@TheCancerMonument.org or at sking@redmagonline.com.

Anna deHaro is a Dallas based radio host and Communications Director of Public Affairs for Clear Channel Radio in Dallas, Texas. She can be reached emailed at Anna@kdmx.com .